INEQUALITIES OF AGING

Inequalities of Aging

Paradoxes of Independence in American Home Care

Elana D. Buch

NEW YORK UNIVERSITY PRESS

New York

NEW YORK UNIVERSITY PRESS
New York
www.nyupress.org

References to Internet websites (URLs) were accurate at the time of writing. Neither the author nor New York University Press is responsible for URLs that may have expired or changed since the manuscript was prepared.

Library of Congress Cataloging-in-Publication Data
Names: Buch, Elana D., author.
Title: Inequalities of aging : paradoxes of independence in American home care / Elana D. Buch.
Description: New York : New York University Press, [2018] | Series: Anthropologies of American medicine : culture, power, and practice | Includes bibliographical references and index.
Identifiers: LCCN 2017044866 | ISBN 9781479810734 (cl : alk. paper) | ISBN 9781479807178 (pb : alk. paper)
Subjects: LCSH: Home care services—United States. | Older people—Home care—United States.
Classification: LCC RA645.35 .B83 2018 | DDC 362.14—dc23
LC record available at https://lccn.loc.gov/2017044866

New York University Press books are printed on acid-free paper, and their binding materials are chosen for strength and durability. We strive to use environmentally responsible suppliers and materials to the greatest extent possible in publishing our books.

Manufactured in the United States of America

10 9 8 7 6 5 4 3 2 1

Also available as an ebook

*To my parents, Ray and Lindy Buch, who cared for me first,
and through it all.*

CONTENTS

LIST OF ABBREVIATIONS

ADA—Americans with Disabilities Act
ADC—Aid to Dependent Children
ADLS—Activities of Daily Living
AFDC—Aid to Families with Dependent Children
CCP—Community Care Program
CHA—Chicago Housing Authority
CNA—Certified Nursing Assistant
DON—Determination of Need
FLSA—Fair Labor Standards Act
HCBS—Home and Community Based Services
HUD—Housing and Urban Development
IADLS—Instrumental Activities of Daily Living
NDWA—National Domestic Workers Alliance
PRWORA—Personal Responsibility and Work Opportunity Reconciliation Act
SEIU—Service Employees International Union
TANF—Temporary Assistance for Needy Families

LIST OF KEY PEOPLE

PEOPLE ASSOCIATED WITH BELLTOWER HOME CARE SERVICES

Maria Arellano—Belltower home care worker, born in Puerto Rico, lived in Back of the Yards neighborhood. Divorced mother of three. Eileen Silverman's care worker.

Debra Collins—Vice President of Belltower Home Care.

Lena Harris—Belltower supervisor, satellite office.

Kathy Hirschorn—Belltower supervisor.

Margee Jefferson—Belltower client. Born in Chicago, lived in Galewood, Chicago. Widow, mother of Bertram (co-resident son) and Ernest (deceased) and two daughters. Grace Quick's client.

Jennifer Martin—Belltower director, satellite office.

Carmen Rodriguez—Belltower supervisor.

Sally Middleton—Belltower home care worker. Born in Central Texas, lived in River North, Chicago. Maureen Murphy's care worker.

Maureen Murphy—Belltower client. Born in Ballinspittal, Ireland, lived in West Lakeview, Chicago. Sally Middleton's client; later Irene Cruz's client.

Doris Robinson—Belltower home care worker. Born in rural Tennessee, lived in Waukegan, Illinois. Mother of Janice and another daughter, grandmother of Teshawn. John Thomas's home care worker.

Carmen Rodriguez—Belltower supervisor.

Eileen Silverman—Belltower client, born and resided in West Rogers Park, Chicago. Widowed mother of Chip (son) and Susan (daughter). Maria Arellano's client.

John Thomas—Belltower client. Born in rural Pennsylvania, lived in Northfield, Illinois. Widowed husband, father of John Jr., neighbor of Linda and Jim Whitting. Doris Robinson's client.

Celia Tomas—Belltower supervisor.

Grace Washington. Belltower home care worker. Born in Gary, Indiana, lived in South Chicago. Married mother of two, primary caregiver of granddaughter Shani. Margee Jefferson's care worker.

PEOPLE ASSOCIATED WITH PLUSMORE HEALTHCARE, INC.

Alicia Morgan—Plusmore trainer.

Ruby Watkins—Plusmore supervisor.

Jackie Wilson—Plusmore supervisor.

Harriet Cole—Plusmore client. Born in Savannah, Georgia, lived in Bronzeville, Chicago. Widowed, lived with brother. Virginia Jackson's client.

Loretta Gordon—Loretta Gordon, lived in Garfield Park, Chicago. Hattie Meyers's care worker.

George Sampson—Plusmore client. Born in rural West Virginia, lived in River North, Chicago. Widowed father of two. Kim Little's client.

Virginia Jackson—Plusmore home care worker. Lived in Hyde Park, Chicago. Mother of two. Harriet Cole's care worker.

Kim Little—Plusmore worker. Born and lived in Garfield Park, Chicago. Divorced mother of two. George Sampson's home care worker.

Hattie Meyers—Plusmore client. Born in rural Alabama, lived in Austin, Chicago. Widowed mother of Brandon Meyers (deceased) and Tommy Meyers (deceased). Neighbor of Rock and Mandy. Sister of Milly, sister-in-law of Arlene. Loretta Gordon's client.

Introduction

On the tenth floor, the elevator dropped Maria Arellano and me off directly across from Eileen Silverman's front door.[1] Maria was Mrs. Silverman's home care worker, I was the visiting ethnographer.[2] Mrs. Silverman, who was in her late seventies, hired Maria to help her live independently. Maria assisted Mrs. Silverman with everyday tasks she could no longer manage alone, like bathing, housekeeping, and running errands. After Mrs. Silverman buzzed someone in to the lobby 14 floors below, she cracked open her door and went about her business, knowing she would hear the elevator doors when visitors arrived. We entered a large beige-carpeted space to the sound of running water coming from the bathroom. On one wall, dark wooden shelves held a television, books, and dozens of photographs. From the back of the room, a bank of windows glowed with a view of Chicago's western horizon. We said quick hellos, setting down our bags. Maria and Mrs. Silverman quickly reviewed their plans for the day, and then Maria excused herself to go prepare Mrs. Silverman's bath.

Mrs. Silverman anticipated Maria's visits for several reasons, but the baths surpassed them all. Mrs. Silverman turned the hot water on a few minutes before Maria was due to arrive each day, filling the bathtub. She liked her baths nearly scalding, but her skin no longer registered the heat as quickly as in the past. A shower was no substitute, Mrs. Silverman told me; a hot bath was the only thing that would calm her nerves and make her feel truly clean. She felt it important that she start the bath herself—she liked to do what she could for herself, to be as independent as possible—even if she no longer felt safe taking the bath without someone else to help her. She needed Maria to make sure the water temperature was safe, and to make sure she did not slip entering or exiting the tub.

To prepare the bath for Mrs. Silverman, Maria used her body to imagine the bodily experience of the older woman. This form of imagination was an exercise in empathy that was as much sensorial as emotional.[3] It was up to Maria to find a temperature that would be warm enough to satisfy Mrs. Silverman's craving for heat without burning the older woman's fragile skin. To cool down the steaming tub, Maria repeatedly drained small amounts of the hot water, replacing it with fresh cold water. As I observed her doing this, Maria gave out a small yelp each time she dunked her hand in the water to open the drain. It was a slow, meticulous process.

In the simple act of testing the water, Maria imagined what it was like to inhabit Mrs. Silverman's body, reaching across differences of age, race, class, and lifetimes of experience to transform her body into a proxy for Mrs. Silverman's older, more fragile, richer, whiter, heat-loving one. Doing so depended on Maria's accumulated experience of what mattered to Mrs. Silverman at a visceral level—which sensations gave her pleasure and made her feel like herself—as well as her intimate knowledge of Mrs. Silverman's bodily condition and limits. When Maria finally got the temperature right, she asked me to test it, and we both agreed that the water was still much warmer than either of us would find comfortable. Mrs. Silverman declared it perfect, and as soon as we left the room, she settled in for a long soak.

In the seemingly mundane act of filling a bath, Maria's subtle attunement and empathy belie common perceptions that home care work is simple, something anyone could do. Officially, home care workers hired through agencies, like Maria, are employed to assist older persons with a concrete list of tasks delineated in bureaucratic documents called "care plans."[4] In these plans, care of persons and care of homes blend into one another. Assistance with bathing, cleaning the bathroom, laundry. Toileting, washing dishes. Grocery shopping, cooking, feeding, cleaning the refrigerator, dressing. This kind of house- and personkeeping work is widely thought of as women's natural inheritance, rather than the consequence of gendered socialization. As a result, there are no national requirements for home care worker training or licensing.[5]

Though technically, Maria was just doing her job, and earning a living, she saw her work as more than the formal list of tasks delineated by Mrs. Silverman's care plan. Her work required more than keeping her client alive. Care also required sustaining her client's way of life, and her subjectivity; her sense of being herself. Maria would later tell me: "Your true self comes out when you're old . . . everyone is a person of their own. And I always try to find that little thing that person likes. They pretty much tell you what their thing is if you give them half a chance, they tell you what their surrounding was, okay? . . . So you find their thing and you work with that."[6] The scalding hot baths were part of what constituted Mrs. Silverman as a "person of her own." Maria never considered replacing Mrs. Silverman's baths with a shower, a more efficient and possibly safer alternative. Jeopardizing Mrs. Silverman's health or safety was also out of the question. Instead, Maria creatively employed a deeply empathic form of bodily imagination to balance between the sometimes conflicting moral goods of Mrs. Silverman's bodily safety and sensorial self-recognition. In balancing between these moral goods, Maria exemplifies the "tinkering" that philosopher Annemarie Mol and her colleagues describe as a "specific *modality* of handling questions to do with the good." The notion of tinkering highlights the ways in which care practices involve practical negotiation and experimentation about "how different goods might coexist in a given, specific, local practice."[7] Home care workers' daily practices involve constant tinkering as they work to realize multiple, and sometimes conflicting, moral goods, such as maintaining their clients' physical health, sustaining their subjectivities, and enabling them to be seen as independent.

Drawing a bath. In this most quotidian of activities, Maria exemplified the subtle bodily attunement that forms an essential part of what the older Chicagoans whom I came to know during two years of fieldwork experienced as good care. Using her body as a flexible medium for reproducing Mrs. Silverman's life, Maria set aside her own emotional and sensory preferences, her own histories of experience, to engage in the intimate life of another. In doing so, she worked not only to sustain her elderly client's biological life, but also her subjectivity and independence. This meant understanding that a searing hot bath was not an incidental pleasure for Mrs. Silverman, but rather a way of sustaining the older woman's ability to feel like the person she knew herself to be.

Home care is one of the fastest growing occupations in the United States.[8] The field is growing due to a convergence of demographic, technological, and social changes. Never before in human history have so many people lived so long. Improved sanitation and new biomedical technologies mean that more people survive the vulnerabilities of infancy and early childhood.[9] Biomedicine transforms previously fatal diseases into chronic conditions, enabling ever longer lives. Yet survivors often require intensive and ongoing treatment. At the same time, declining fertility rates, the expansion of wage labor, and changes in family organization mean that there are fewer people in younger generations available to provide care for older adults who require it. In places like the United States, where elder care was traditionally the province of unpaid female kin, women's increased participation in wage labor markets further strains previous methods of organizing care for frail elders. A variety of market-based forms of long-term care have emerged to fill this gap. Market-based long-term care is provided both in institutional settings like nursing homes, as well as in settings like assisted living facilities and private homes. Home-based care is increasingly preferred because it enables older adults to remain more independent.

Few older adults and families are able to afford extensive and ongoing long-term care, and most rely on either private insurance or public programs to fund it. As the population ages, increases in the overall public spending for home care have been inadequate to meet demand for these services. In the United States, many older adults rely on the federal health programs Medicare and Medicaid to fund long-term care. Medicare provides federal health insurance to older and disabled adults, but only funds ongoing care in nursing or private homes for limited periods of time in the aftermath of acute health events. Medicaid, a social health care program for people with limited resources, is administered by the states. Medicaid provides ongoing long-term care, and funds the vast majority of home care services.

Cash-strapped state Medicaid programs play a significant role in determining home care wages. Pressures to keep taxes low incentivize policy makers to reduce spending on programs like home care. In most states a greater number of older adults are eligible for publicly funded home care than can be provided by current budgets, leading to long waiting lists. As a result, state programs aim to provide as much service as possible without expanding budgets, which creates pressure to keep home care wages low. Yet low wages make it difficult to recruit and retain workers with the empathic and domestic skills necessary to sustain older adults' homes and independence. Consequently, these programs face immense economic and workforce challenges as the number of people requiring care continues to grow.

Home care workers like Maria play an essential role in the everyday lives of older Americans, but they struggle to live up to societal expectations of independence. Home care workers' wages and working conditions place them squarely in the ranks of the working poor. Home care jobs are disproportionately filled by women of color and immigrant women. Their wages are constrained, in part, by older adults' limited budgets and by limited public funding for their services. In 2015, home care workers in the United States earned an average hourly wage of $9.61. Very few home care workers work full time due to the unpredictable hours and part-time schedules common across the home care industry. Thus, median annual wages for home care workers in 2015 were approximately $13,000, having remained stagnant over the previous 15 years.[10] Home care workers rarely receive health insurance, paid sick leave, vacation pay, or retirement benefits through their jobs. More than half of them live in households with incomes low enough that they qualify for a variety of public poverty-relief programs.[11] Thus, a similar proportion of home care workers live in households that rely on public benefits including food stamps, Medicaid, and heating assistance to make ends meet.[12] Because of their use of need-based government benefits, home care workers, like other members of America's working poor, are regularly depicted as lazy, as not contributing their share to the social good, and as inappropriately dependent on public largesse.

Home care work is often considered in tandem with other "direct care" jobs in which workers are responsible for the daily labor of sustaining life, like bathing, toileting, and feeding older and disabled adults. Some direct care providers are employed in institutional settings like assisted living facilities and residential care programs for people with disabilities. Direct care workers with Certified Nursing Assistant (CNA) training are qualified to work as nursing home assistants and home health aides. These forms of employment pay slightly higher wages than home care, but face similar challenges. While home care workers sustain the lives of vulnerable older adults, their economic status is closer to that of maids and housekeepers.[13] Housekeepers, child care workers, and home care workers share the designation of being (at least partly) domestic labor. The low wages earned in these types of jobs reflect, in part, the ways in which the broader economy depends upon the invisibility of exploited labor hidden within the walls of American homes.

Paid care work sits at the nexus of two of the United States' biggest social challenges: rising inequality and an aging population. Policy and advocacy initiatives typically treat poverty and care of the aged as distinct forms of vulnerability. They are considered as having separate causes that require different solutions. For this reason, perhaps, people have often asked me whether this book focuses on older adults or on care workers. By attending to the lives and histories that coalesce at the urgent intersection of aging and inequality, I argue that these challenges are bound up with one another. At the heart of this book lie the diverse relationships generated by care and their connections to longer national histories, policies, and institutional contexts. The vulnerabilities of older adults and care workers are commingled: low wages and poor working conditions render workers' lives precarious. In turn, high turnover rates and endemic worker shortages translate into waiting lists and lower quality care for older adults. In home care, the fate of older adults and the working poor are connected, entangled by the broader indifference of a society that devalues both aging and care. Poverty is generated in tandem with care.

Centered around quotidian moments like Mrs. Silverman's bath but also within the longer life histories and social contexts that shape people's lives, this book argues that everyday care work is a form of generative labor that simultaneously sustains independent persons and intensifies inequality. By generative labor, I refer to the wide range of moral imaginings, practices, processes, and relations through which people work together to generate life in all its forms. I focus on care relationships in practice; that is, on the historical and everyday processes that create home care relationships, and the meanings and consequences of these relationships for those who directly participate in them and for society. And I attend to the ways in which these relationships are embedded in peoples' longer histories of experience and in institutional contexts. In turn, home care relationships themselves constitute persons, histories, and institutions. In the process of making life happen, practices of generative labor like home care create forms of meaning, personhood, morality, relatedness, and difference. Care also generates inequalities that are defining features of social life in the United States.

By focusing on home care as one form of everyday care, this book lays bare the contradictions that animate care of all kinds in the United States. Home care shares much in common with other occupations responsible for the daily labor of sustaining domestic life and the lives of vulnerable people across the life course. Ideologies of caring labor being something other than "real work" have long been formalized by legal and regulatory structures in the United States, legitimizing and exacerbating intersecting forms of economic, racial, and gender inequality. Though generally discussed separately, the history and fate of domestic workers, child care workers, and care workers who attend to both disabled and older adults are connected. Each of these groups undertakes labor that has long been considered women's duty to perform, unpaid, on behalf of kin. These fields are shaped by ongoing legacies of gender and racial discrimination such that they are dominated by women of color and immigrant women. While some of the challenges facing paid home care are unique to the field, the daily care provided by care workers makes possible all other economic activity. In return, these workers are paid so little that they and their families live in perpetually unstable and precarious conditions. In a nation founded on a belief in political and personal independence, we struggle to accommodate the profound interdependencies that make life possible. Those who care for the most vulnerable among us become ever more vulnerable themselves. It is a system that consumes those who sustain it.

Nobody Really Cares

Many months after my lesson with Mrs. Silverman's bath, Maria and I sat down for a formal interview. More than any of the other home care workers I got to know, Maria had taken me seriously when I asked her to treat me like a trainee during my weekly visits with her and Mrs. Silverman over the previous eight months. She teased and cajoled me until I could finally perform the simplest tasks in a way that mimicked her finely attuned care. At the grocery store: "No, don't push the grocery cart—let Mrs. Silverman push so she can lean on it if she gets tired." At the library: "Don't suggest books to her unless they have it in large print font—if you say the book is good, she will check it out, but if she can't see the words she gets frustrated and gives up—then she won't have enough books to last the week."

Maria spent the afternoon caring for another client before the interview. She was visibly exhausted, smiling, and trying to be upbeat. We had not seen each other for a few weeks before the interview. As she caught her breath and I tested my recorder and microphone, we chatted a bit, catching up on each other's lives. Maria had come to terms with the idea that her husband, who had moved out of their apartment a few months earlier, was not coming back to her. She was planning to move to a new, smaller basement apartment that would cut her commute time in half, and she had no special affection for the gritty Back of the Yards neighborhood where she had lived for several decades. Named for the stockyards and slaughterhouses that once drew generations of immigrants, and an epicenter of early twentieth-century labor and community organizing, Maria experienced Back of the Yards as dirty and dangerous.[14] She thought the leafy, calmer North side would be better, though it meant leaving behind the places that reminded her of her son, who had died a few years earlier. It would be a fresh start—not a chosen one, but maybe one that would work out for the best.

When Maria turned the conversation to me, I tried to deflect, but empathic as always, Maria could tell that I was feeling down. My eyes welled up. The previous evening my parents had called and told me that my father had been diagnosed with Parkinson's disease. My pain was fresh and shallowly disguised. Maria immediately knew this for what it was. She put her hand on my shoulder and I struggled not to melt into my sadness. Maria did not press me to talk more, and I turned our attention back to the interview, finding reprieve in the dry legalese of consent forms.

I started the interview by asking Maria to tell me the story of how she became a home care worker. The words falling into the tape evoked heartbreak, struggle, and survival. Raised by her grandmother in Puerto Rico, Maria was sent to live with her mother in Chicago as an adolescent. They moved constantly, her mother worked long hours and went out most nights. When her younger brother came to live with them, things took a turn for the worse. Maria ran away to Texas with her boyfriend as a young teen. He drank too much and worked too little. Eventually, she left him. By her mid-twenties, Maria was raising their three children on her own. She learned about jobs in home care from another mom at the public aid office.

She started as a home care worker soon after, joining the rapidly growing ranks of women earning near-minimum wages caring for others. "I don't know how we managed, but I always had food to feed my children. Always. It didn't matter if I was inventing. Take a few hot dogs, some salad and you literally had supper. People would say, you have nothing to eat. I said, yes we do. We have macaroni or just a big pot of white rice and ketchup, but we had food. . . . There were a few things that would hurt. My children would say 'is there any more?' and I would be eating. I would say 'oh no. But I am full. Here.'" She shook her head, remembering the hunger.

Maria narrated this memory as another lesson in caregiving, describing how she made it through days as tough as the one I was having. "I try not to let it show with my patients. If you live long enough, you deserve so much. As a caregiver, you are so happy, you show everyone such a good time that nobody even noticed where you lacked." She continued, "But you also need laughter! I very strongly believe you can be crying your head off, but as soon as you walk out the door, wash your eyes, put a smile on your face. My problem is not yours. Don't ever, ever forget that, okay?" I responded that this sounded exhausting, and Maria grimaced. "It is exhausting. I remember, I took care of a lady. She was blind and I was going through a lot. I would cry and she could not see me. She'd ask, "how are you doing?" "Oh, I am just fine." But it was exhausting. It was better though, because I could cry, cry all day with her 'cause I knew she could not see me. It was a relief that I could cry. I wasn't around the kids. I wasn't able for her to see me losing it. I was going through so much, you know. But you put your face on. And I put my face on for a long time."

Like other home care workers I knew in Chicago, Maria wore her smile like armor, protecting herself and those around her. Maria's smile is an instance of what sociologist Arlie Hochshild calls "emotional labor." A defining feature of service work, emotional labor requires workers to manage their affective performances in order to elicit particular emotions from consumers in ways that benefit corporate bottom lines.[15] While Hochschild argues that emotional labor alienates workers from their true emotions, home care workers like Maria were critically aware of the distinction between their own subjectivity and the ways they expressed emotion around clients. Home care workers' emotional labor was intentional and protected older adults from being accountable for the ways that their independence is bound up with their care workers' hardships.

The moral demand for carers to set their own needs and feelings aside in order to sustain the lives of others is at the very heart of the social relations that generate both independence and inequality. Maria's smile was a professional mask shielding her frail and vulnerable elderly clients from sharing in her suffering. In her insistence that "my problems are not yours," Maria acknowledged that American ideologies of responsibility and independence held her alone responsible for her circumstances—even though many of her struggles were directly connected to low wages, long hours, and unpredictable schedules that created the conditions in which she cared for others. These ideologies were formalized in the employee handbook of the home care agency that employed Maria, which listed discussing "your personal problems with your client" as one of the "unprofessional behaviors" that could get a worker fired. Sharing problems could lead to workers and clients becoming overly enmeshed in one anothers' lives. The irony was not lost on Maria: she was responsible for her own struggles, even though her clients' most intimate problems had become her responsibility. The paltry wages she was paid to make her clients' problems her own may have been necessary for her survival, but they did not compensate for the lack of reciprocity in the terms of her home care relationships.

Maria also wore her face to protect herself from the indifference of others. She spoke of teaching her kids "the strength you have to have. Everybody can feel sorry for you, but nobody is going to hold your hand. And the same thing with yourself. Everybody loves you, and cares for you, but nobody wants to hear you say I am a hundred dollars short for my phone bill. But that same person will invite you out to eat and spend two hundred dollars on your dinner tomorrow. But would he give you that hundred dollars? No." In Maria's experience, the pity, concern, and affection of others had never translated into the actual assistance she needed to support her family.

She continued the lesson, telling me how she used her emotional labor not only to please her clients, but to protect herself from their hollow concern. "You learn to swallow it, take care of it. Deal with it, give a little if you can. You don't have to give a hundred percent, but you could show a hundred percent. Okay? One day, you might forget to fix the bed, or throw out the garbage, or give that extra hug or something because your mind was somewhere else. That day, that week, your world is coming down. Like yours. You know. You can give me twenty-five percent, fifty percent, but show one hundred percent. Because even though everybody will feel sorry for you, nobody really cares. And that's the secret of staying alive in America."

A damning statement, even more so from this woman, this mentor of mine who had spent her adult life caring for people in every direction—her children, her husband, her elderly clients. How to reconcile Maria's profound commitment to caring for others, and her indictment that "nobody really cares"? Rather than interpret her statement as an admission that her own care was insincere, I interpret Maria as commenting on the way her life was shaped by flows of empathic attunement and concern that only ran in one direction—from her, and care workers like her, to those they served. In Maria's experience, those for whom she cared at work were more concerned with the ways in which her emotional performances affected them than with her actual well-being. So she used her smile to camouflage the exhaustion and absent-mindedness produced by the unrelenting strain of economic and social precariousness. For Maria, a woman deeply committed to caring, survival demanded accommodating society's fundamental indifference.

The secret to staying alive in America, Maria argued, was never forgetting that society expected her—and workers like her—to be materially independent. No one would offer to pay her bills no matter how much they enjoyed her companionship. No matter that her same skillful companionship, in the context of paid labor, was so poorly compensated that it rendered her life and the life of her family perpetually precarious. Care workers enable their clients and employers to be seen as independent and make it possible for higher paid workers to sustain their households and families while still earning sustainable livelihoods. Nevertheless, public discourse in the United States often represents low-wage workers, including care workers, as parasitic, dependent on public largesse rather than as crucial contributors to national well-being.[16] The irony of being seen this way was not lost on Maria, who underscored how odd it was that so many could rely on her caring labor and still think of her as problematically dependent because of her economic status. Maria's generative labor was only worthy of state-subsidized compensation if framed as independent "work" caring for non-kin. On the other hand, receiving state support for similar kinds of labor performed on behalf of her family rather than consumers represented an unacceptable form of dependence.

The indifference Maria experienced is connected to America's foundational ideology of independence. It refracts through people's experiences and stories of care, shaping the ways that they care for one another and the ways that this generative labor produces gradients of care, concern, and indifference. Ideologies of independence create erasures and silences that make secret the profound ways people—in this case older Chicagoans and home care workers—are necessary to one another. In laboring to maintain older adults as independent persons, care work simultaneously generates a seemingly compulsory veil of indifference that conceals the profound contributions and hardships produced by care labor. Social indifference to care workers' struggles feeds off of and intensifies broader forms of racial, gender, and class inequality. The indifference demanded by ideologies of independence is the secret at the heart of care that generates inequality in the very moments that sustain life.

Generative Labor

Through the concept of generative labor, I analyze how care can simultaneously produce forms of morality, independent persons, and social inequality. This concept highlights two aspects of social life: first, that the everyday practices that make and sustain life—both social and biological—are necessarily entwined with the makings of political economy. In this sense, these practices are labor. Second, these forms of labor determine which and how different lives matter around the world; they generate both lives and social difference in the process.[17] The category of generative labor highlights the messy, disparate forms of practice through which people work to make life happen, and how these practices continually bring particular kinds of persons, social relations, and political economies into being. Generative labor draws attention to the ways in which these practices do not simply reproduce unequal social structures, but create kinds of inequality and difference that are historically connected to but also distinct from those of previous moments.[18]

Analyzing care as one of many vernacular forms of generative labor draws attention to the ways in which different moral understandings of human interdependence are created and put into practice, as well as to the political and economic social forms that are generated through those practices.[19] By theorizing care as generative, I argue that we should understand it as a central force in creating social life.

The concept of generative labor builds on the concept of reproductive labor, crucially extending its insights across the life course and to new questions. Sociologist Evelyn Nakano Glenn defines reproductive labor as "the creation and recreation of people as cultural and social, as well as physical human beings."[20] Feminist scholars have long theorized care by thinking of it as reproductive labor, showing how social relations of care reproduce existing forms of difference and inequality. The concept of reproductive labor highlights the ways in which capitalism devalues social interdependence and the daily labor necessary to sustain social life. But the language of reproduction has several limitations. Its implied link with biological reproduction has led scholars to emphasize child-bearing and childrearing, limiting theorization of the care across the life course. The language of reproduction also implies that such labor has the effect of extending past and present ways of living, including social inequalities, into the future. I argue that the labor of creating social and biological life does not simply extend already existing forms of sociality, it constantly generates both life and ways of living.

As conceptualized by feminist scholars, reproductive labor complements and makes possible the "productive labor" by which people create goods and services for market exchange.[21] Historical gendered divisions of labor under industrial capitalism rendered productive labor the more highly valued province of men. Capitalist markets typically do not account for the costs of reproducing laborers' lives when accounting for the costs of making things.[22] Divisions between productive and reproductive labor are enforced when government policies deny public and corporate responsibilities for sustaining people's lives.[23]

The persistent devaluation of reproductive labor in capitalist economies partially fuels paid care work. Critical feminist scholars have long argued that women's responsibility for unpaid reproductive labor in domestic spaces is at the heart of women's oppression, and a primary driver of intersecting racial, gender, and economic inequality.[24] It is not surprising that women who have privilege and resources tend to hire others to do the most belittled forms of reproductive labor—the "dirty work" of maintaining homes and human bodies—while reserving for themselves the more morally and emotionally valorized aspects of childrearing and elder care.[25] Throughout the history of the United States and other colonial/postcolonial societies, poor women of color have been coerced into undervalued reproductive labor through chattel slavery, occupational discrimination, and racially restrictive labor laws.[26] These racial divisions of reproductive labor in the United States are, as Glenn writes, "key to the distinct exploitation of women of color and is a source of both hierarchy and interdependence among white women and women of color."[27]

The coercive recruitment of poor women, and especially women of color and immigrants, into paid reproductive labor generates what anthropologist Shellee Colen calls "stratified reproduction." This term describes the processes by which different groups come to have vastly different resources to support their physical and social reproduction as a result of intersecting social differences based on class, race, gender, ethnicity, ability, migration status, etc.[28] Processes of stratified reproduction themselves reproduce inequality by, according to anthropologist Marcia Inhorn, "inequitably privileging the reproductive trajectories of elites over those of the poor and disempowered, whose right to reproduce may be called into question and even despised."[29] Though the language of reproduction directs attention toward biological reproduction and early life, these forms of labor sustain life at every age.[30]

Many analyses of the devaluation of reproductive labor in capitalist societies focus on the ways in which capitalism demands but does not compensate the labor of reproducing new generations of workers. By focusing on the reproduction and care of young people, calls to "invest" in the "future" uncritically accept the ways that capitalist economies value the future over the past and productive capacity over all other ways of valuing life.[31] Capitalism's demand for productivity is intertwined with American anxieties about aging and obsessions with independence. As people age and move away from playing "productive" roles in the paid workforce, they come to be seen as "dependent" and are treated as marginal to society. Older Americans, who may need help with daily activities, come to be considered as burdensome, drawing the energy and resources of younger generations away from productive activities.[32] I use the term generative labor to advance an intersectional, life course approach to thinking about the stratification of labor that sustains social and biological life.

Drawing on the thinking of the Gens Collective of feminist anthropologists, the concept of generative labor attends to people's "varied pursuits of being and becoming particular kinds of people, families, or communities." These scholars argue that political economic forms like late capitalism are derived from "divergent life projects" and thus are not unified logics but rather "unstable, contingent networks" that are fragile, intimate, and "generated from heterogeneity and difference." From this perspective, analysis of political economy requires attention to "the full range of productive powers and practices through which people constitute diverse livelihoods (and from which capitalist inequalities are captured and generated)."[33] The Gens approach links the apparent diversity and complexity involved in the daily generation of life to the production of global economic forms, specifically contemporary capitalism.

I also advance the category of generative labor as a means to enable comparison between Euro-American practices of "care" and the myriad other social practices and moral imaginaries through which people around the world engage with the interdependent practices that make life possible.[34] Generative labor both expresses and generates peoples' moral imaginaries about which kinds of persons and social relations exist and should be supported. Moral imaginaries provide the social and moral basis upon which systems of resource distribution are justified; as such they play a crucial role in the generation of political economies like capitalism. In contrast to similar concepts like "ideology" or "belief," I use the concept of moral imagination to highlight the social processes that generate shared but diverse ideas about how life should be lived.[35] While the term "imagination" implies a focus on cognitive processes, I use it expansively to include the ways in which bodily practices produce moral understandings.[36] Moral imagination draws attention to the dynamic ways people play with, work on, and adapt their ways of thinking about what "should be" through ongoing engagements with one another and over time. These engagements crucially include the intertwined practices of care, memory, and storytelling through which people come to understand humans' interdependence on one another and the broader world. Attention to the ways generative labor is mutually constituted with moral imagination shifts focus from normative discussions of care toward a focus on how people understand, make sense of, organize, and practice interdependence as a foundation for sociopolitical-economic life.

When scholars use the term "care" to describe a wide variety of practices around the world, they often do so in ways that uncritically reflect powerful moral imaginaries that inflect the term care with connotations of warmth, concern, and kindness.[37] Both popular and academic discussions of care often index Euro-American moral imaginings about the ways that the interdependencies necessary for generating life should be organized—who should care for whom, in what ways, for which reasons, and to what extent. These assumptions infiltrate both scholarship and popular discussion of care. Clearly identifying how moral imaginaries shape the ways that researchers and everyday people in the United States (and elsewhere) describe care is an essential step toward more meaningful analyses of the ways that generative labor creates different kinds of lives and political economies.

Euro-American moral imaginaries about care, kinship, and work are often described as the "separate spheres" ideology, which prescribes distinct and gendered moral, relational, and affective norms for the public and private spheres. The ideology that public and private are "separate spheres" plays a constitutive role in capitalism, historically arising alongside and naturalizing the movement of paid work out of dwelling places (where agricultural, manufacturing, and human reproduction occurred in close proximity) and into designated workplaces like factories. The public sphere of work and politics, long associated with men's sociality, is imagined as a sphere of autonomous, rational individuals who appropriately act in self-interested ways. The private world of intimate relations, associated with women, has been constructed as a sphere requiring intimacy, solidarity, and sacrifice to reproduce and sustain social relations.[38] Separate spheres ideologies imagine money and love as morally opposed motivations for human action, and especially for care.[39]

The implicit association of care with sentiment and moral practice diverts attention from the crucial role that the care plays in generating different kinds of persons and political economies. Imagined as inherently private, care is paradigmatically found in bodily intimacies between mothers and children, and thus evokes notions of domestic warmth, attachment, love, and sustenance. These associations make it difficult to think of care as a source of violence or suffering; the term is often used in ways that excise or romanticize the physical pain, exhaustion, and exploitation that many carers experience. Moral imaginaries that oppose economic and sentimental motivations make it difficult for many Americans to imagine that care could be appropriately provided within economic markets or by state institutions. In this formulation, good care is that which is undertaken by those motivated by deep moral and emotional commitments to the well-being of others rather than by material and economic concerns.[40] Thus, professionalized and market forms of care like health care, child care, and paid home care suffer suspicion from an implicit contrast between the warmth of familial love and the assumed sterility, bureaucracy, detachment, and economic incentive associated with clinical and institutional settings.[41] Care, when understood as principally referring to loving kin practices, impugns the labor and motivations of paid care workers who, some worry, might take these jobs "just for the money."[42]

Scholarship that uncritically adopts dominant Euro-American moral imaginaries surrounding care hinders analysis of the darker aspects of care, including the ways that care practices produce power and inequality in social life. A growing number of ethnographies show how the implication that care is an inherent moral good obscures practices of power operating in the name of care. Instead, these ethnographies suggest that investigations of generative labor should ask questions about how different understandings of "the good" implicate specific forms of power and violence. For example, anthropologist Lisa Stevenson documents the ways in which the Canadian government's attempts to care for indigenous people with tuberculosis valued life itself, as measured by epidemiological population counts, over actual lives and indigenous ways of life. These forms of care created intergenerational disruptions and violence, which contribute to high rates of youth suicide. Current forms of care through suicide prevention continue to value life itself over the ways of being that are dreamed of and pursued by indigenous youth.[43] In a different vein, anthropologist Angela Garcia shows how forms of attachment and care among kin can simultaneously participate in harm and violence. In this case, mothers and daughters in the Hispanola region of New Mexico care for one another by participating in shared heroin use as a form of solidarity, relief, and affection in the midst of long histories of dispossession, poverty, and the absence of other forms of communal and governmental care.[44] In France, anthropologist Miriam Ticktin shows the perverse effects of that nation's attempt to care for international victims of sexual assault and HIV by offering them asylum. Ticktin argues that the purportedly apolitical morality of this form of care instantiates a violent politics that disregards the suffering caused by global economic inequalities and forces migrants to perform various forms of victimhood.[45] In each of these cases, we see how the language of care can obscure forms of violence and how practices called care can themselves perpetuate violence and inequality. Thus, instead of narrowly understanding care as a form of nurturance or moral response to suffering, thinking about care as a form of generative labor helps to direct attention to what such labor produces—including violence.

The concept of generative labor highlights the ways in which moral imagination, interdependence, and social inequality are generated over and over, in new and not-so-new forms, in the same intimate moments and processes that generate life. It opens analytic possibilities for recognizing the transformative as well as reproductive potential of those inevitable moments of friction that occur amidst the messy day-to-day of making life happen. Considering care as not only reproductive but generative draws attention to the processes that create generations of people and regenerate complex social forms, highlighting that which is altered and made anew through these processes.[46] From this perspective, the fact that care is deeply patterned by racial, class, gender, age, and global economic inequalities is not simply a legacy of discriminatory history but is central to contemporary processes generating both personhood and social relations.

Home care and other forms of paid care are especially important forms of generative labor in that they are multiply generative—making possible the lives of older adults, workers, and their respective families. Home care also makes possible the broader workings of an economy that depends on inexpensive care to make available other workers for more highly valued and lucrative occupations. The contradictions and entanglements created by the concurrent, multiple forms of generativity in paid care highlight the links between multiple scales of care from the intimacies of embodied interactions to the abstractions of national policies.

Generating Independent Persons

In the United States, independence is socially valued. Widespread ways of morally imagining how independence is constituted play a central role in the ways that people, institutions, and governments organize interdependence. Despite Americans' emphasis on independent living, people of every age and ability profoundly rely on others.[47] We rely on other beings—both human and non-human—in every aspect of life, from those activities necessary for our very survival to those that form the foundation of our ways of life. Older adults' independence comes into question not because they are more reliant on others than those of other ages, but because their interdependencies are more visible. In the United States, concerns about independence index the forms that interdependent relationships take, with anxiety accruing to moments and forms of reliance believed to impede individuals' abilities to make decisions without being influenced by others. I show that independence is not a quality that Americans gain outside of their relationships with others, but rather is generated within relationships characterized by difference and inequality.

Independence is a normative category rather than a descriptive one. In the United States, independence is a defining moral criterion for personhood—meaning a recognized member of human social worlds.[48] Most of the older adults I knew in Chicago saw meeting normative expectations of independence as an ongoing battle of attrition fought in subtle and everyday ways against the mounting age-related debilities changing the ways they inhabited the world. Failing to live in a manner deemed "independent" might mean that others no longer recognize them as full persons and instead treat them as children or objects who are unqualified to make the most basic decisions about their everyday lives. In the United States, the attribution or denial of independence is often coterminous with the attribution of personhood.[49] To be seen as dependent is to be seen as something less than a full person.

This form of personhood, sometimes described as the "liberal person," is enshrined and inscribed in US laws, social policies, and economic systems. Anthropologist Elizabeth Povinelli describes liberal personhood as based on the moral claim that "what makes us most human is our capacity to base" intimate, political, and economic relations "on mutual and free recognition of the worth and value of another person rather than basing these connections on, for example, social status or the bare facts of the body."[50] Liberal personhood also prioritizes the ability of individuals to live in a manner that reflects and expresses their subjectivity; this is sometimes described as freedom. In this ideology, freedom is made possible by independence.

For many older adults in the United States, continuing to live in a private residence (rather than in an institution) is one of the most important markers of their ongoing independence and personhood, regardless of how much assistance they require from others to do so. This reflects the fact that in the United States, a person's ability to exert agency and autonomy in daily life is widely understood (and legally enshrined) as intimately tied to control over homes and private property. In order for private ownership of property to make sense, people must be seen as autonomous and distinct from the social relations in which they are embedded, such that one individual human can be seen as having rights over possessions.[51] Euro-American legal and philosophical traditions connect notions of the person and independence to an individual's rights and abilities to control houses and other forms of private property.[52] For example, US legal theorist Margaret Radin has influentially argued that certain kinds of property, such as homes, are constitutive of personhood and that control over these objects is critical for psychological well-being.[53] Working within these widespread forms of moral imagination, prominent US-based gerontologists John Rowe and Robert Kahn have argued that successful aging and independence are defined in part by "continuing to live in one's own home, taking care of oneself."[54] The centrality of independent living to notions of personhood thus creates particular risks for those who struggle to maintain private homes due to bodily or economic limitations.

One of the generally unacknowledged contradictions of liberal personhood is that presuming that persons have value outside of their social relations devalues the actual relations and forms of obligation that generate such persons.[55] Especially in physically vulnerable moments, generative labor plays a critical role in making, transforming, and unmaking persons—liberal or otherwise. At the beginning of life, forms of generative labor, including feeding, bathing, and cooking, play central roles in the constitution of personhood around the world. Toward the end of life, the social relations that arise through generative labor as people experience dementia, brain death, and vegetative states often create liminal, situational, and contested forms of personhood. For such people, everyday care practices can play a significant role in generating or eroding personhood.[56]

Home care generates older adults as independent, liberal persons even as home care workers' very presence threatens to reveal elders' diminishing ability to meet the demands of liberal personhood. Together, home care workers and older adults navigate these fraught relationships, working to arrange themselves in ways that obscure older adults' dependencies. Older adults recognized themselves as independent not only when they were able to make autonomous decisions, but also when they were able to act as equal partners in reciprocal relations and maintain familiar ways of life. Enabling older adults to remain "a person of their own," as Maria put it, also meant caring for them in a manner that recognized their diverse subjectivities by creating social and sensorial continuity in their lives.

Concealing older adults' dependence means effacing the most complex and nuanced aspects of care workers' jobs. These practices exacerbate perceptions of home care as unskilled labor, and conceal home care workers' vital contributions. Such concealments are facilitated by workers' social marginality; their contributions are simultaneously naturalized and hidden by their gender, their poverty, and their race. Though home care workers sustain older adults' personhood and enable their residential stability in later life, their jobs do not enable workers to similarly create stable lives for themselves or their kin. Home care policies and practices presume that workers are less vulnerable than their clients. Moreover, home care practices generate older adults as liberal persons in part by indifference toward care workers. From this perspective, independence is generated by inequality.

Independence as Policy in the United States

In the United States, ideals of liberal personhood and independence guide the advocacy efforts and social policies fueling the home care industry's rapid growth. Notably, these efforts typically focus on the independence and personhood of older and disabled adults, but have less to say about low-wage workers, who are also made vulnerable by liberal capitalism. On the other hand, critics of social safety net programs mobilize ideologies of independence to undermine programs that support poor families by arguing that such programs harmfully promote dependence.

Since the 1960s, disability rights advocates have mobilized discourses of independence to fight the institutionalization of disabled and older people in places like asylums and nursing homes. Disability rights activists imagined deinstitutionalization as a mechanism of liberation, in which inhumane institutions were replaced by a continuum of community-based supports. One of the movement's signature policy victories, the 1990 Americans with Disabilities Act (ADA), requires that services for people with disabilities are provided in the most appropriate, community-integrated setting possible, rather than in institutions. The ADA explicitly frames independence, and especially independent living, as both a civil right and a method of reducing the costs of dependence and institutionalization.[57]

Beginning in the late 1970s, neoliberal health care reformers recognized the potential cost savings gained from deinstitutionalization, which shifts many costs of daily care (like food and shelter) to individuals and their families. For example, when the Illinois state government established its state-funded home care program, called the Community Care Program (CCP), in 1979, it described the program as "aimed at assisting seniors to maintain their independence and providing cost-effective alternatives to nursing home placement."[58] Implementation of deinstitutionalization has long been entangled with efforts to shrink public funding for social services, leaving inadequate community supports and shifting the costs of care to individuals and families.[59] As the population of older adults has grown in the intervening decades, the twin goals of supporting elders' independence and reducing the costs of elder care have only become more urgent priorities for state and national policy makers.

Deinstitutionalization led to policy reforms expanding public funding for Home and Community Based Services (HCBS), accelerating the expansion of the home care industry. At the federal level, this was accomplished primarily by making Medicaid funds available for home care and other HCBS. As one measure of the growth of HCBS, in 1995, only 18 percent of Medicaid long-term care spending went to HCBS. By 2013, 51 percent of all Medicaid long-term care spending went to HCBS services. In 2013, about half of the older adults receiving long-term care funded through Medicaid were living at home rather than in institutions.[60]

The relationship between home care work and poverty is not coincidental. Many home care workers, including Maria, found home care jobs through welfare-to-work programs created by neoliberal welfare reform policy in the 1990s. Many home care agencies participate in these programs and receive tax incentives to hire welfare-leavers. Based on charges that welfare encouraged dependence, welfare reform ended the practice of providing funds for single mothers to care for their own children on charges that welfare encouraged dependency. Welfare reform pushed a vast pool of women into dead-end, low-wage jobs by placing limits on the total length of time they could receive benefits and by making those benefits contingent on their participation in job training or welfare-to-work programs.[61]

At the same time, policy makers aiming to restrict government spending on health care programs like Medicaid fail to allocate the funds necessary to pay care workers living wages. Care workers' labor enabling older adults to remain in their homes is accompanied by their own economic and housing insecurity. Thanks to low wages, rising housing costs, and limited public support for low-income housing, home care workers—like other low-wage workers living in major cities—often struggle to afford housing, food, and other necessities. In Chicago, as elsewhere in the nation, the twin goals of cost-effectiveness and independence generate home care practices and policies that undermine the stability of home care relationships and intensify social inequality.

Ideologies of independence create impossible expectations for older adults and for home workers. Both kinds of people experience societal indifference when they struggle to meet social expectations that they sustain impossible forms of independence. Workers' and older adults' related struggles to be recognized as liberal persons shape the intimacies of paid home care in profound ways. In home care, older adults and working-poor women, two groups marginalized by American fixations with independence, are thrown together. They depend on one another to stay alive, and to make those lives meaningful.

Studying Home Care in Chicago

I moved to Chicago in 2006 to learn from and with those involved in the city's home care industry. Nicknamed "the city of broad shoulders," Chicago has long been imagined as a city shaped by (implicitly white) male manual laborers and industrial workers employed by Chicago's factories and famous (but now mostly defunct) slaughterhouses, lumberyards, and rail yards.[62] Later, images of Chicago's dangerous and crumbling public housing projects dominated portrayals of the city. The projects became symbols of violent young black men trapped in neighborhoods without jobs and of the dependence of unemployed single black women on a neglectful society.[63]

Chicago's position as the gateway to the American West has made the city a major center of both national and international labor migration.[64] Since the early 1900s this legacy positioned Chicago as one of the most important laboratories for urban ethnography and scholarship on the social geography and reproduction of race and inequality. The majority of these studies have focused on urban life within Chicago's famous ethnically and economically segregated neighborhoods, attending less to the ways in which movements between such neighborhoods influence the texture of urban life.[65] As care workers spend time in households across Chicago's racially and economically segregated neighborhoods, they experience and embody its inhabitants' diverse ways of life. Focusing on home care work draws attention to the ways in which domestic and direct care workers, primarily women of color, have long knit the city together, crossing between homes and neighborhoods.

The experiences of home care workers in Chicago highlight the contributions that poor women of color have made to the life of the city. Home care is one recent instantiation of the hierarchies of race, class, and gender that have organized labor in Chicago for more than a century. The city was created not only by the backbreaking and bloody work of manual laborers but also by the care labor of generations of domestic workers. The legacies of gendered labor and racial segregation that shaped the city are remade anew as home care weaves together the lives of the city's elderly with those of its poor.

Chicago is a critical node in webs of care that link the fates of workers and families across the city, the country, and the globe. Sociologists including Arlie Hochschild and Saskia Sassen use the term "care chains" to describe the processes that draw women of color from the global south to wealthy northern cities where they care for the young, sick, and elderly members of richer, whiter families. Frequently, poorer women and kin in the global south are then drawn from rural areas to expanding cities to care for the young and old relatives of migrant care workers.[66] I follow anthropologist Laura Heinemann in describing neighborhood, national, and international linkages between women and families as "webs of care," to account for "the multidirectional flows" of care that create interdependencies implicating people, families, and communities across great distances.[67]

Some scholarship describes care chains as a relatively recent consequence of globalization. Yet in Chicago, these linkages stretch back at least to the Great Migration of black Americans who came North seeking to escape poverty in the Jim Crow South in the early- and mid-twentieth century.[68] Pushed into domestic service jobs by discriminatory laws and practices, many of the black women who came to Chicago could find employment only as domestic workers. Today, as then, transnational immigrants join the daughters and granddaughters of Chicago's Great Migration as both groups are funneled into poorly paid domestic work and direct care jobs.

Home care in Chicago is patterned by the city's unique history and social geography. Yet long legacies of both migration and racial segregation shape labor markets and family life around the country. No one city or region can represent the vast diversity of the United States, or any practice or population within it. At the same time, home care in Chicago shares much in common with home care as it is practiced around the country. In many ways, the state and local policies regulating home care in Chicago are unremarkable—funding is neither especially generous nor stingy, and regulations are not significantly more or less demanding compared with other regions.[69] In some cities, immigrant workers fill a greater proportion of direct care jobs than in Chicago. In many rural areas, direct care workers are more likely to be white.

The experiences of home care workers and older adults in Chicago are theirs alone. Yet in their very specificity, these experiences offer a sense of the diverse hopes and struggles of people working to stay alive and to make their lives meaningful. Nationally, gradients of inequality and the desire for independence pattern social relations. As economic inequality rises, working-class families of every stripe have seen their wages stagnate.[70] The decimation of social welfare programs pushes people into low-wage jobs that do not cover the costs of food and housing, much less the costs of child and elder care that people might provide for kin if they were not working multiple jobs to keep roofs over their heads. All the while, the costs of care—the costs of sustaining life—rise. Everywhere older adults and families face impossible choices about how to fund and provide care, choosing among limited and mostly undesirable options. Across the United States, people feel powerfully their obligations to provide for those they love. They seek work that is both materially and morally rewarding, hoping their labor will sustain their families and contribute to their broader worlds.

Chicago's webs of care forge human links among the city's otherwise segregated populations, as home care workers provide care across economic and racial spectrums. As in much of the United States, Chicago's home care services are bifurcated along economic lines. If older adults (or their kin) have sufficient income and assets to afford to hire workers themselves, they have a number of choices about how to organize this care. They can hire workers directly on what is colloquially known as the "grey market"—a clever term referring both to the typical color of elders' hair and to the legal ambiguities introduced by hiring workers directly.[71] Others rely on full-service home care agencies that employ and supervise home care workers. Not surprisingly, most of Chicago's privately funded agencies were located on the wealthier, whiter, north side of the city and served the city's northern and western neighborhoods and suburbs. At the time of my research, privately funded agencies were subject only to the rules and regulations applied to other businesses in the state.[72]

In Chicago, older adults who have limited assets and income can receive services through the Illinois Community Care Program (CCP).[73] The CCP negotiates contracts with home care agencies to provide publicly funded services to older adults who qualify. Agency contracts spell out supervisory ratios, training requirements, and hourly reimbursement rates for home care. While the CCP pays for most of the cost of care, older adults receiving its services typically pay a small sliding-scale fee for services (usually less than a dollar per hour of care). In Chicago, many of the CCP-funded agencies' offices are located in and around the downtown loop and serve clients across the city. The city's privately and publicly funded home care services are connected through webs of interdependence. For example, an older adult's children might pay for a home care worker to make sure their parent doesn't fall, while the home care worker's parents rely on CCP services.

The fieldwork upon which this book is based involved traversing domestic and bureaucratic sites of care across Chicago from 2006 to 2008. I spent much of that time learning from the employees and clients of two home care agencies: Plusmore Home Care Inc., and Belltower Senior Services. In the following discussion, I note the costs and wages in 2008, and in parentheses adjust these numbers to account for inflation as of 2017. However, reimbursement and wages in the intervening years have not kept up with inflation: accounting for inflation, workers earned slightly less in 2017 than they did the decade prior.

Plusmore Home Care Inc. provided need-based services to approximately 2,500 older adults through its contract with the CCP. The state reimbursed Plusmore approximately $13 ($14.71 in 2017) per hour of care it provided, which exceeded its total costs (including insurance, bonding, and administrative overhead) by only pennies per hour.[74] The huge economies of scale generated by Plusmore's large caseload enabled it to turn a profit on these small hourly margins. Plusmore workers were represented by the Service Employees International Union (SEIU), which negotiated contracts and advocated with the state government to increase wages. Plusmore workers earned a starting wage of $7.65 ($8.66 in 2017) an hour and received a five-cent raise each year they remained employed up to a maximum of $9.15 after 26 years of employment. Notably, these wage increases were not adequate to keep up with inflation. Plusmore's supervisors, workers, and clients were overwhelmingly black women; the agency also had designated supervisors and workers able to serve Spanish- and Russian-speaking clients.

Belltower was privately funded, serving about 200 clients who paid an average of $19 ($21.50 in 2017) per hour of care.[75] At the time of my fieldwork, Belltower paid workers a starting wage of $6.75 ($7.64 in 2017) per hour. While some benefits and paid leave were available at each agency, very few workers qualified for them.[76] Although the gap between fees and wages was far greater at Belltower, administrators worried constantly about generating enough revenue to keep the organization running. Belltower's clients were nearly all older white adults, while its workers were most likely to be African American, Puerto Rican, or Filipina. Belltower also employed a sizeable number of Polish and West African women.

During fieldwork, I spent several months in each agency's offices, observing supervisors' daily work, training sessions, and staff meetings, and in the process learned about hundreds of older adults and workers beyond those I was able to observe directly. I also collected a wide range of institutional policy documents, recordkeeping systems, and promotional material. I joined agency administrators when they attended meetings of local professional groups and attended meetings at the local SEIU offices, learning about new trends in elder care as well as state and national policy advocacy undertaken by these groups.[77]

I worked with agency supervisors to identify and seek permission from older adults and workers willing to allow an ethnographer ongoing access to their homes and lives. Older adults who required live-in care or had significant cognitive deficits were excluded from the study due to concerns about their ability to provide ongoing consent to my presence. Supervisors tended to direct me toward clients whom they perceived would be welcoming, based on their own interactions with older adults. Plusmore supervisors additionally seemed to screen out clients living in situations in which they believed I would not be safe. After older adults consented to participate in the study, I sought separate consent from their workers.[78]

The heart of my ethnographic fieldwork was the six to eight months I spent visiting the homes of each older adult when their worker was present. The older adults with whom I conducted this intensive participant observation included five women and two men; the workers were all women. Demographically, both older adults and workers reflected the general population of their respective agencies. Older adults received anywhere from eight hours to more than forty hours of care each week. This group reflects somewhat healthier and perhaps lonelier older adults than the home care population at large, given that these older adults were willing to let me encroach so much on their lives.

I visited home care pairs on a weekly or biweekly basis, depending on their schedules. Each pair had its own daily routine, and with each I developed methods of balancing my time with them. Most older adults and workers spent about half their time doing activities together, and half their visits separate from one another. Typically, when a home care worker was cleaning or cooking, the older person sat in another room. I moved between them—sometimes alternating during the same visit, sometimes balancing things out over different visits. When sitting with older adults, we chatted about matters light and heavy—family and neighborhood gossip, politics, times gone by. I asked workers to treat me as a trainee, showing me how to do their jobs and allowing me to assist with daily work ranging from grocery shopping to cooking to cleaning. With only one older adult was I invited to help with bathing and dressing. Some workers were more interested in my help and attention, while some were warier—their invitations more than anything else determined how I spent my time. As we worked, they told me of their lives past and present, their families, and their dreams. They teased me for my apparent lack of a personal life and wondered why I was bothering them instead of keeping busy caring for my own ailing grandparents. Asking for instruction as a carer-in-training elicited a wide variety of moral and practical instruction about what they considered "good care." I regularly joined workers and clients in running errands, eating in restaurants, and attending doctors' appointments. At the end of six or eight months of visits, I sat down and recorded long life history interviews with these workers and older adults, asking them to tell me about how experiences of care had shaped their lives.

Over time, most (thought admittedly not all) workers came to see me as a pleasant and helpful companion. This is not to say that my relatively elite status and relationships with supervisors receded into the background. Some participants came to see me as a potentially useful ally, occasionally asking me to advocate with supervisors and others on their behalf.[79] Many workers hoped that by participating in this project, audiences both near and far might come to better appreciate their labor. In this way, my arguments are both animated and limited by older adults and home care workers' broader moral and personal projects.

Organization of the Book

This book moves across social and temporal scales, engaging home care as involving both the immediate practices and relations that develop in the course of daily care and the longer histories of care, training, and policy that give shape to daily practice. People's past experiences of care form their subjectivities and moral imaginations, thereby playing a crucial role in shaping the stakes and practices of home care. Drawing on extended life histories and observations, the first chapters show how past experiences of care and kinship shape the stakes of care. Home care management and training practices harness these legacies of care and transform them into paid care work. The later chapters focus on the ways in which everyday home care practices work to sustain older adults' bodies and homes and in the process strive to engender independent persons who live "on their own." These chapters show how home care practices simultaneously hide the traces of workers' labor and forestall emergent forms of reciprocity. Workers embody the very different subjectivities of those for whom they care, generating embodied moral hierarchies that deepen and recreate the social inequalities that pattern home care. While these practices generate older adults as independent persons, they simultaneously generate instability in the lives of both workers and elders.

The first chapter draws on the life histories of three very different older adults. In telling their histories, older adults' narratives describe how their moral imagination of care, personhood, and kinship were formed. These forms of moral imagination are crucial for understanding the meanings and stakes of care for older adults and how they distinguish good care from bad. Crucially, older adults did not imagine independence as requiring them to sustain their lives without assistance from anyone else. Instead, many understood independence as generated through reciprocal relationships in which they contributed equitably to the well-being of those upon whom they relied. Older adults typically took solace in the fact that their home care workers were paid, seeing this as a more independent manner in which to receive care than relying on unpaid but morally obligated relatives. In this way, home care kept older adults from becoming a burden on those they loved, protecting them from the always present specter of dependence.

Home care workers typically develop indispensable expertise caring for kin in difficult circumstances. Drawing on the life histories of two home care workers, chapter 2 shows how workers' care for kin generates forms of moral imagination in which care practices are inextricably linked to notions of obligation, reciprocity, and sacrifice. For workers, these moral and domestic lessons become survival skills thanks to long histories of discriminatory social policy that regenerate the racial and gendered contours of poverty while funneling poor women of color into domestic and care jobs. Their stories highlight their resilient and creative responses to poverty, and their central role in generating the independence of others.

Home care agencies transform women's domestic expertise and their moral imaginations into wage labor that can be bought and sold at an hourly rate. Chapter 3 traces the extractive process through which publicly and privately funded agencies train, staff, and manage the workers and clients necessary to their enterprise. By making care into work, agencies strive to manage the fraught tensions that regularly arise in home care, all the while navigating contradictions at the heart of American ideologies of public and private. Agencies face competing pressures to stay afloat, abide by relevant laws and public policies, be good employers, and provide high-quality services. Home care agencies and their supervisors negotiate the contradictory demands of care ideologies, economic pressures, and legal regulations in order to generate both profits and lives. In the process of navigating these competing demands, home care agency practices generate older adults and home care workers as independent both from one another and from the broader kinship networks and histories in which they are embedded.

Embodied care practices are at the center of home care work. They generate deep but fragile entanglements between the lives and bodies of older adults and those of their home care workers. These practices involve forms of empathy that blur the boundaries between older adults' and home care workers' bodies and their personhoods. Chapter 4 shows how home care workers engage with their own bodies as the experiential ground for imagining and sustaining elders' lives. In the process, they transform seemingly straightforward tasks like cooking, cleaning, or grocery shopping into moral practices that help older adults feel independent—like the persons they have always been. Through this process, home care workers' bodies become the ground upon which moral hierarchies between persons are built, experienced, and justified on a day-to-day basis. Daily home care practices generate ways of embodying social hierarchies, and shape individual subjectivities, thereby making those hierarchies feel morally legitimate.

Taking care of homes is inseparable from caring for persons in home care. Chapter 5 shows how homes are invested with history and memories, becoming a material sign of older adults' independence. In tandem with maintaining elders' bodies, workers learn to maintain their clients' homes to sustain their personhood. They attend to the smallest details, noting where to place each kitchen item or bottle of soap so that an older adult will be able to find it. They also gently suggest subtle changes to the home to make it safer or more inviting, drawing on their knowledge of elders to figure out what changes will be palatable. Flows of people, money, and material goods link workers and elders' homes. Agency policies attempt to restrict these flows, leaving workers struggling to maintain their own households. In this way, home care workers' domestic instability is generated by the same policies and practices that generate older adults' abilities to live independently.

By the end of my fieldwork, three of the workers that I knew best had quit or been fired from their jobs; another seemed on the verge of leaving. In each case, job loss stemmed from workers' inabilities to sustain both their own households and those of their older adults without blurring the boundaries between them. Across the United States, home care faces perpetual worker shortages and endemically high turnover levels estimated at between 60 percent and 90 percent per year. Chapter 6 examines cases of turnover in rich ethnographic detail, focusing on the ways in which the inability of agency and public policy to recognize the interdependence of older adults, workers, and their families contributes to this startling statistic.

Current forms of care generate inequality through efforts to sustain independent persons. The conclusion builds on key arguments of the book to suggest several routes toward building a caring economy that instead generates equitable interdependence. Current methods of organizing care leave people and families across the social spectrum with inadequate and precarious ways of sustaining ever longer life spans. The growing demand for care only exacerbates these challenges. Continuing to undervalue generative labor while placing its demands on the backs of those already struggling is simply untenable. Instead, I invite readers to imagine with me ways of organizing care work that value familial histories and embodied labors so as to sustain meaningful ways of life. Valuing care work is a crucial step toward generating a society that values people of every age and background.

Generating Independence

Older Adults' Life Histories

George Sampson was a slim man, his face and limbs all sharp angles exaggerated by the fastidiously pressed slacks and dress shirt he wore each day. A widower with one child living out of state and two more nearby, he lived alone in a small one-bedroom apartment in one of the Chicago Housing Authority's (CHA) buildings for seniors.[1] His asthma and diabetes had become debilitating about five years before we met. He decided he did not want to move in with any of his children despite his increasing frailty. After a series of hospitalizations, his children had begged him to move into their homes. He said, "I could have moved in with my daughter or Junior or gone to West Virginia. They would come and get me. I had so many offers, you know. They still want me to." He even tried staying with them after a particularly serious illness, but "They was wearing me to death. I couldn't have no privacy. They would be up all day, all night. If they're not asleep or something, they be upstairs or downstairs, where ever I decide to be, and be there. 'You need so and so. You need so and so.' They'd call themselves helping." He rolled his eyes with that last phrase, remembering his exasperation.

Instead, his home care worker Kim Little visited him each afternoon. She made sure he ate a healthy lunch, she prepared a warm supper, and kept his apartment immaculately tidy, the way he liked it. Without Kim, Mr. Sampson struggled to keep his blood sugar steady. He told me he hoped the arrangement would last the rest of his life: "If I can't do for myself then I don't know if I would want it then. I wouldn't want no one to worry about me. No way. As long as I can do something, I'm okay. I've been doing for myself ever since I was five or six. It's just habit. I ain't helpless, you know."

Like many of the older adults I knew in Chicago, Mr. Sampson felt his life balanced precariously at a kind of crossroads between the independence of "doing for myself" and an unknown, unwanted future relying on kin. Mr. Sampson had served in World War II and once worked three jobs to support his family. Now he was too frail and sick to manage on his own but was reluctant to be supported by kin. Like many older Americans, Mr. Sampson believed that concern, effort, and goods were supposed to flow from parents to children. He worried that if circumstances reversed this flow, he would burden his descendants.[2] Older Americans' anxieties about burdening younger generations also reflect their fears that they will lose control of their daily lives and become subject to their children's (and others') concern and interference.

Many older adults prefer care from paid workers, seeing such care as supporting their independence and sustaining their autonomy. The wages home care workers are paid for their caring labor help older Americans to see themselves as equal participants in market exchanges, rather than dependents whose care is the product of coercive intergenerational obligations. For older Chicagoans, remaining independent did not require them to sustain their lives entirely on their own. Rather, older Chicagoans viewed themselves as independent so long as they could contribute equitably in relationships with those upon whom they relied. Home care became a kind bulwark against the possibility of becoming a burden, and a source of hope against the looming threat of dependence.

Older adults' concerns about sustaining independence reflect the central role this value plays in dominant American conceptions of personhood. I follow a long history of anthropologists in conceiving of personhood as a culturally and historically variable category of membership in social worlds. Understood this way, personhood is socially made and unmade, through daily practices which are shaped by cultural understandings that vary considerably across space and time. Personhood and subjectivity are bound up with one another, in that individuals' sense of who they are and their preferences are formed by their experiences, including broader social understandings of personhood.[3] Recognizing or refusing the personhood of particular beings has profound consequences. These include determining which kinds of beings are able to participate as full members of communities and polities.

In common US discourse, the notion of a person is synonymous with individual members of the human species. American debates about personhood (for example around abortion or corporation rights) often presume it to be a binary status: either a being is or is not considered a person. In practice, chronological age, work history, citizenship, marital status, race, sexuality, and gender all factor into the ways that individual humans are formally recognized as persons in the United States. For example, citizens over the age of 18 are granted the right to vote; at that age male citizens are currently required to register for the draft. Eligibility for federal retirement programs like Social Security depends on a person's citizenship, age, and work history.

Around the world personhood is understood quite differently, and those differences help to reveal some taken-for-granted assumptions about personhood in the United States. Across contexts, attributions of personhood allow for gradations of difference encompassing the variety of social roles and experiences related to a being's membership, status, and relationships in communities. These attributions are fundamentally relational, meaning that beings are recognized (or not) as persons through social relations, rather than prior to these relations.[4] Understandings of personhood are also profoundly moral; they reflect and generate expectations of those who participate in social life. I use the awkward phrase "beings" because, in some places, personhood is attributed to ancestors, spirits, plants, animals, and features of the landscape as well as to living human individuals.[5] For example, in New Zealand, the Wanganui River was granted status as a legal person after 140 years of advocacy and negotiation by the indigenous Maori Whanganui iwi (kin group), who consider the river an ancestor.[6] Even the term "beings" limits our understanding of personhood because in a number of contexts, personhood accrues not to individual beings, but to multiple socially connected beings. For example, in many countries, including the United States and Argentina, business corporations are granted status as legal persons.[7] Personhood is sometimes denied to humans for reasons including problematic paternity, disability, race, and age.[8]

Personhood is a dynamic status, emerging throughout the course of social life. Social understandings of personhood also change in concert with social and technological change. The concept of personhood encompasses changing roles and statuses over time; it is made and unmade through relations that change over each person's life course. Beings who fall outside of local age- and gender-related norms (as well as norms related to other kinds of social difference) are likely to find their status as persons threatened.[9] For example, in the United States young adults gain legal rights of citizenship on the basis of chronological age. However, in many American communities, people are socially considered full adults once they establish households that are physically (and ideally financially) separate from those of their parents. Economic and social conditions that hinder young people's ability to live independently thus also threaten their status as full adult persons. Maintaining a household is a key marker of personhood in the United States; it is thus no surprise that older adults fear bodily changes that threaten their ability to live under their own roofs.

Across the life course, experiences of care generate people's understanding of their own personhood and that of others. Most obviously, the ways that people care for others reflect whether those others are recognized as full persons. For example, in the United States, care of a pet might signal that the pet is considered a particular kind of person—a family member, but not an autonomous individual. Similarly, care for children often signals that they are persons-in-becoming—biologically human individuals who do not yet have the developmental or social capacities to function as fully independent persons. More subtly, experiences of care play a key role in socializing people to particular ways of morally imagining what a person is, how persons are expected to behave, and how interdependencies between people should be organized.

Normatively, full adult persons in the United States are thought to exert autonomous agency in the world according to the dictates of their will, which requires that they are mentally, physically, financially, and domestically self-determining and self-sufficient. From a young age, children in the United States are taught to perform these forms of self-sufficiency, often through practices that obscure the central roles parents—and especially mothers—play in producing these performances.[10] Children increasingly gain roles, status, and rights as they are able to perform greater physical and financial self-sufficiency, in part because their reliance on others becomes even less visible. Older adults, on the other hand, fear being unmade as adult persons and treated like children if they are seen as less self-sufficient. Older adults who have begun to acknowledge their need for assistance thus find themselves in a precarious position, defending their status as full, independent, adult persons.

This chapter examines how older Chicagoans articulated evolving understandings of care, personhood, and independence as they narrated their life histories to me.[11] Older adults' narratives show how their models of liberal personhood arose in the context of these diverse life histories. Across their stories, experiences of care and family, work and hardship intersect with experiences of race, class, and gender.[12] Discourses of independence weave through their specific histories. This shows how dominant discourses are interpreted through life experience and come to shape people's moral imaginations. The differing understandings of personhood that older adults develop across their long lives played a central role in how they thought about and evaluated care.

A Sense of Independence

The stroke she suffered two years earlier had knocked Harriet Cole for a loop. She did not talk about it much with me, except to emphasize that now she could do nearly everything she did before it happened. She credited her determined independence for her recovery. She told me, "When I first got sick, they said, 'You need someone to push [you] in the wheelchair.' I said, 'Oh, hell, no. Everybody is going to be busy.' I got in the wheelchair myself and pushed the wheelchair and got all over the house by myself. You got to maintain a sense of independence." Even so, Mrs. Cole agreed when the hospital social worker suggested that she get a home care worker funded through the CCP program. It was nice to have some help around the small, pristine two-bedroom apartment she shared with her brother. The small co-pay she was charged each month empowered her. She did not see herself as dependent on Virginia Jackson, her home care worker. Mrs. Cole saw herself as the younger woman's boss.

Mrs. Cole's determination to remain independent seeped into nearly every aspect of her life. As a black girl growing up in the interwar years in the South, she learned early that she could easily be treated as less than a person because of her age, race, and gender. Mrs. Cole also learned that wealth and property could gain a person status and respect in a racist world. She learned that material prosperity created both care and protection. From these early experiences, Mrs. Cole came to believe that others would treat her as a person only as far as she was able to reciprocate any material or social support she received. She ferociously defended her property as the material guarantee of sustained independence. For her, independence was not defined by an absence of relying on other people, but rather by arranging those interdependencies in the right ways. She believed a person achieved independence through sustained reciprocity, by never being in anyone else's debt.

Despite the stroke, Mrs. Cole insisted she was very much the same person. Her watchful, proud presence commanded respect. Her dark skin glowed, showing only a few lines despite her more than 80 years. She was svelte and somewhat shorter than the five feet eight inches she told me she had once stood. Many days, she welcomed me wearing the clothes she wore to the building's exercise class that she had attended earlier in the morning, always apologizing for not having had time to change. Even then, her hair was perfectly coifed, her face recently made up, and bright red or coral lipstick freshly applied. She kept her home fastidiously too. The apartment was a study in white—gleaming white linoleum tile, freshly painted white walls, and all white furniture. Two cream-colored upholstered chairs with gilded wood trim sat empty along one wall of the room, protected by shiny plastic covers. A handsome dark wood cabinet along the back wall held a small television, framed photographs, and a few plants absorbing light from the tinted window above.

About three years before we met, Mrs. Cole's husband died. Shortly thereafter, Mrs. Cole and her brother moved to their small two-bedroom apartment in one of the Chicago Housing Authority's subsidized buildings for seniors. She sold most of her furniture. The pieces that had once filled their grand 15-room home were too large and ornate for the utilitarian apartment. When I was not helping Virginia, I sat and chatted with Mrs. Cole at the white Formica table that sat near her small galley kitchen. She spent most afternoons at the table watching her favorite courtroom television shows.

She encouraged those around her to develop the independence she had spent a lifetime cultivating, regularly offering Virginia and me advice on how to make sure we never became dependent on anyone. It was a lesson taught in a thousand ways. At Christmastime, Mrs. Cole told Virginia not to get her any gifts but instead to get something nice for Virginia's boyfriend because "I don't matter to you, but he does. Spend your money on him—he helped you move into that third-story apartment because you need him. You have to do things for those that are nice to you, because that's what keeps you independent." Even though she had help around the house, Mrs. Cole implied, she remained independent because she was able to reciprocally help the people who took care of her. Mrs. Cole imagined independence as the absence of moral and economic debts, as the freedom to do as she pleased because she did not owe anyone in the making of her life.

The link between material security and independence was a lesson Mrs. Cole learned early. Raised near Savannah, Georgia, she was the middle child of nine. Mrs. Cole remembered sharing a bed with her grandmother, her father's mother, when she was very young. The family moved to Gary, Indiana, when she was still young. Her father worked in the mills and cleaned a doctor's office at night. She was grateful for his hard work, saying, "We grew up in nice surroundings. Everything we had, we had from him. Everything that came out new, we had. I don't know if you remember, ice cream rolls, when they first started bringing that out, we had that. And malts. And the big containers of ice cream, he'd bring those home. He took us to shows. My dad took good care of us." Mrs. Cole's father gave her one example of what care might look like: working hard so you could provide nice things for those who relied on you.

Mrs. Cole learned that those who earned a lot of money also earned respect and independence. As much as she admired her father's hard work, as a girl Mrs. Cole dreamed of following in her Big Mama's (her mother's mother) footsteps. Big Mama was rich and beautiful, but she did not rely on anyone else to provide for her. At the time, Big Mama was one of the only people selling insurance in her small Southern town. Mrs. Cole never forgot the power of Big Mama's reputation, which allowed her a modicum of freedom despite the entrenched racial caste system that limited the movement of the other black people in town. She recalled, "I always wanted to be like her because she always had tons of money and whatever she wanted. She always sent us money. Her house was the first one in the area that had all indoor plumbing and everything. It had a pond in the front yard with goldfish in it. She had an organ upstairs and chickens in the backyard and a fig tree. I would climb that tree and eat figs for days." She continued, "Remember, black folks in those days, there were all kinds of things we couldn't do down

South. I remember once visiting Big Mama, I wanted some ice cream so I sat at the counter, and my auntie told me 'You can't sit there.' The store lady said, 'well, that's Ms. June's granddaughter so she can sit there.' She had such a reputation in that town." Wealth and a reputable job, Mrs. Cole learned early, could enable her to transcend the life circumscribed for black women.

Mrs. Cole started working at a young age and learned quickly that she was expected to support those who supported her by contributing part of her wages to her family. As a young girl, she babysat for the neighbor and then worked in a drugstore. She remembered that "whatever I made, I gave part of it to the household. When I came home from the drugstore flashing five ten-dollar bills, my mother said 'come over and sit,' and snatched one of the bills." Mrs. Cole continued, "Ever since then, I gave back to the household. It teaches independence and something you want to do for yourself to do better." In Mrs. Cole's narrative, her mother forcibly required her to contribute to the household upon which she depended. This obligatory reciprocity, Mrs. Cole argued, was central to her learning how to be an independent person.

After finishing high school, Mrs. Cole moved to Chicago and went to a business school where she learned secretarial skills. During these early years in Chicago, Mrs. Cole lived in the Phyllis Wheatley home, a communal residence for young, unmarried, working, African American women.[13] Residents lived four to a room and shared a kitchen with the whole house. Rent was cheap, maybe 50 cents a week, which was about all she could manage since she was sending money home to her parents. It was hard making ends meet while earning so little. Living in tight quarters, Mrs. Cole learned that she would have to protect the little she had. For example, Mrs. Cole told me of the time she suspected one of her housemates was drinking her milk from the communal refrigerator, so she poured milk of magnesia into it. The next night, the woman became violently ill. When the emergency personnel asked if she knew what happened, she told them, "Well, if she'll admit that she stole my milk, I can tell you what happened. But if she didn't take my milk, then I don't know nothing about it.'" Telling the story, Mrs. Cole repeated that line over and over, laughing and concluding, "She never stole my milk again, that's for sure!" Mrs. Cole freely shared her income with her family, seeing this as a fair exchange for the many years her parents had supported her. But she would not suffer those who helped themselves to her few hard-earned things. Those who failed to reciprocate, or even worse, those who took from her without permission, showed a parasitic dependence that she defended herself against.

Mrs. Cole also learned that if she wanted to have control over her life, she was going to have to earn the things she wanted for herself. She worked for a department store and then a law office. She soon realized that "everything I was doing was related to insurances, so I took the test. And then, selling insurance. As long as a customer kept their policy, I got a little check. It taught me independence." She told me, "I like the good things. I always had some girlfriends, who I thought were sharp and nice, but they were not independent people. One friend had a boyfriend at *Ebony* magazine. He was very nice to her, I thought. I took her to a Christmas party one night down at a lawyer's office. Every two seconds she had to stop and call him. I thought, 'I don't want this kind of life.' The heck with that. That's crazy. I never wanted anybody because of what they had. That's good. That's yours. I want to get my own. If you're going to talk to me, have a job or some kind of career builder or do something for yourself. I liked my own independence." Mrs. Cole saw that if she could not reciprocate the generosity of others, she would not be able to define the terms of her relationships. She demanded that those with whom she associated be similarly independent.

After many years selling insurance, she met her husband at church and married him soon after. She never spoke much about him except to say that he had been kind, godly, and successful. After they married, she moved into her husband's home in Bronzeville. Once a flourishing, wealthy black neighborhood, the city had neglected it for years by then. The Coles furnished the house luxuriously and enjoyed entertaining friends from work and church there. Mrs. Cole fondly remembered their three aggressive guard dogs, who successfully kept watch over the house and deterred both criminals and neighbors from visiting. Mrs. Cole and her husband were fiercely protective of the house, a sign of their social standing amidst an increasingly threatening neighborhood.

Mrs. Cole narrated her life as a classic American Dream story in which she achieved prosperity through hard work and self-reliance despite the challenges posed by her race, gender, and working-class roots. As Mrs. Cole told stories about defending her property—sometimes violently—I'd often catch a glimpse of Virginia, working out of Mrs. Cole's line of vision, with an expression of shocked abhorrence on her face. Mrs. Cole was not easy to like—she was suspicious and unapologetic, even when telling stories about causing others pain. The ferocity with which Mrs. Cole protected her possessions always struck me as telling of more than the idiosyncrasies of her personality. Her pride and defensiveness were also signs that she felt her hold on prosperity and the independence it bought remained precarious.

Moving into subsidized senior housing threatened Mrs. Cole's sense of independence after so many years spent closely guarding her property. In these new surroundings, she struggled to protect her possessions and reconstruct the material security that made her feel independent. Though she no longer had a high fence and terrifying dogs to protect her home, she creatively fashioned new barriers. She liked that her new apartment was more than a dozen stories up. Even more, she liked that visitors had to show the security guard identification before they were allowed on the elevators. Mrs. Cole demanded that visitors remove their shoes and wash their hands and made Virginia and me do so repeatedly when we went back and forth between her apartment and the basement laundry. She was suspicious of her new neighbors. She refused to interact with them and sprinkled borax powder around the perimeter of her apartment, creating a chemical barrier to the pests she feared they harbored. It was uncomfortable to be sharing a building with precisely the sort of people from whom she had spent a lifetime trying to distinguish herself.

Similar anxieties fed Mrs. Cole's apprehension about having a home care worker. She thought people willing to do such low-paying jobs were likely to be those who were lazy and "didn't want to make something better for themselves." Mrs. Cole's care worker Virginia was also a black American, but their shared racial background did not earn Virginia any extra sympathy from the older woman. For Mrs. Cole, the hardest part of having someone come into her home was "to trust them. I don't trust nobody. I laid things around the house purposely to see if they would take them. I'd leave money around and my watch. One worker came to my house and she had been drinking." When I asked Mrs. Cole what she thought people should know about having home care workers, she told me that the most important thing is that "they should watch their home.

Everybody is different. You watch your stuff. You cannot have people have free reign over what is yours. You got to watch. You wouldn't let me come into your home and not know where I am going. That wouldn't make sense, right? But there are people who don't watch stuff. You got to keep it together. That makes a difference."

Mrs. Cole's need to let untrusted care workers into her home deepened her sense of vulnerability. In other ways, having a home care worker helped to minimize the threats that old age posed to her sense of independence. Since her stroke, Mrs. Cole admitted that she no longer had the stamina to clean as vigorously as she would have liked. Home care workers helped make up the difference, maintaining her home and possessions in the way she desired. The first home care worker Plusmore had sent, right after the stroke, had been her favorite because "she was really clean. She'd clean the bathroom and do different things. You'd never have to worry about it . . . She did some things I didn't think about doing. It was like when I was in the big house, I had a service come over and do housework with me." Mrs. Cole narratively erased the many changes that had occurred since her husband had died by comparing her home care workers with previous housekeepers. According to Mrs. Cole, a good care worker was one who maintained her home and hard-won middle-class lifestyle, both signs of her independence.

Mrs. Cole minimized her growing reliance on others and her diminished means. Instead, she emphasized the ways in which she still cared for herself and others. Mrs. Cole spoke of her relationship with Virginia as one of mutual benefit rather than dependence. She said, "I definitely take my shower. At 5:00 I'm fixing my brother's breakfast and then I make up my own bed and I get everything together. Like I told Virginia, 'I don't leave things around just because you're coming here. You only come two days a week. These things I'm going to do whether you come or not.' I said, 'Don't think that's why I want you here. You're not doing that much.'" Mrs. Cole emphasized that she was not dependent on Virginia's help, but rather saw her care worker's labor as a kind of luxury available to her because she could afford the CCP's required co-pay.

Mrs. Cole presented herself as her care worker's generous patron, countering any implication that receiving care made her dependent. She told me repeatedly about the small gifts she regularly gave Virginia, enacting her advice that independence could be maintained by reciprocating assistance. For example, when Virginia moved to a new apartment, Mrs. Cole gave her hand-me-down throw pillows and other decorations she thought Virginia might like. She gave Virginia a paid day off for her birthday, signing the younger woman's time sheet but telling her not to come in to work that day. For Mrs. Cole, these kinds of reciprocity, as well as her financial ability to purchase services, were a way to show that she was still a valuable and independent person despite stroke-induced debilities.

Like so many of the older adults I met in Chicago, Mrs. Cole's narrative focused on the continuities across her life and minimized the ways in which her life had changed. Comparing home care workers to domestic servants was one of the ways in which Mrs. Cole maintained her sense of being a middle-class person against the bodily, domestic, financial, and social vulnerabilities she faced in later life. Mrs. Cole's experiences of care early in life had formed her understanding of what it meant to be a person, shaping how she lived and how she evaluated home care. In a racist and sexist world, black women were treated as full persons only when they could wield power and status derived from incontrovertible material wealth. For Mrs. Cole, being an independent person meant engaging in ongoing material reciprocity—sending money to the family that raised her, paying wages, and giving gifts to care workers. Independence did not mean absolute self-reliance, but rather having the material resources necessary to reciprocate any assistance she required.

Not a Piece of Furniture

The air outside Maureen Murphy's apartment shimmered with record-breaking heat much of the summer I spent with her. Every news outlet harped on the dangers posed by the 100+ degree temperatures, and city officials pleaded with Chicagoans to check on elderly kin and neighbors to avoid a repeat of the deadly heat wave that had killed hundreds a decade earlier.[14] Ms. Murphy no longer had anyone to check on her, save Sally Middleton, the home care worker she had hired through Belltower a year or so earlier. Ms. Murphy's apartment, a second-floor walk-up in a leafy neighborhood on Chicago's north side, was warm but not sweltering. It bothered Ms. Murphy to keep the small window air conditioner running—the machine was noisy and drowned out the sound of the nearby church bells by which she marked her day. She kept it on anyway, intimately aware of the risks heat posed from her decades working as a nurse. Ms. Murphy kept the shades drawn across the long bank of windows that stretched across her modest apartment, blocking the hot sun.

Ms. Murphy spent most of her life caring for others, first as the foster daughter and eldest child in a large family in rural Ireland. Later, she worked as a nurse. These experiences gave her a different perspective on care and personhood than many older Chicagoans. For Ms. Murphy, care generated and sustained personhood through careful attunement to an individual's social history and related sensory preferences. From her point of view, independence was not so much about moral and material freedom but instead about being treated as a unique individual with particular sensibilities.

Most days, I found Ms. Murphy sitting at the big dining room table that crowded her apartment's doorway. Sitting on a foam pillow so she could see over the table to the small black and white television she kept tuned to sitcom re-runs, Ms. Murphy's legs barely reached the floor. Ms. Murphy never struck me as frail, despite her small stature and her constant pain. Her hands were gnarled and frozen into claws by rheumatoid arthritis. Though slow and ever mindful of her balance, Ms. Murphy moved around her small apartment with firm purposefulness, her dark eyes lit with an even mix of determination and humor. We got along right away—her warm, thick Irish accent, ever-ready gallows humor, and matter-of-fact loneliness immediately endeared her to me. During each of my weekly visits I sat with Ms. Murphy, helping the older woman sort through the jumbled disarray of papers, bills, rubber bands, used Kleenex, and office supplies spread over the table. Each week, we searched for the checkbook she perpetually misplaced. No matter how tidy the table was when I left in the evening, the next week I found it returned to chaos.

As we sat, Sally scurried around in the back of the apartment, cooking Ms. Murphy's supper, laundering the towels, and tidying up the bathroom. Sally occasionally asked when Ms. Murphy would be ready to eat but otherwise moved through the apartment with brisk, quiet efficiency. After more than a year caring for Ms. Murphy, Sally had a seemingly intuitive sense of what the older woman wanted. She knew to make sure the milk and yogurt in the fridge were fresh, how much salt Ms. Murphy liked in various recipes, and that she liked the sheets on her bed tucked in as tightly as possible. She and Ms. Murphy still sometimes disagreed about how many items should be out on top of the dresser. Ms. Murphy liked all her jewelry, medicines, and trinkets visible, but Sally thought the mess just made it harder for Ms. Murphy to find things. Sally generously showed me how to cook Ms. Murphy's favorite dishes—Irish style beef and potato stew and the mashed potato and cabbage dish called Colcannon. She learned these recipes when she first started working with Ms. Murphy. The ingredients were similar to the stews she had cooked for her aging parents during the decades she spent caring for them in central Texas, but she had learned the subtle differences in the Irish recipes that Ms. Murphy preferred. The two women, both white, were about 15 years apart in age and both were marked by their accents as transplants to Chicago.

In just over a year, Ms. Murphy's rheumatoid arthritis had become so painful that she no longer left the apartment alone. As soon as the weather turned cooler, she began asking me to accompany her for short walks. Usually we made it only a block or two, pushing her walker past the back of the large Catholic church she had attended regularly for decades. No matter how painful, she told me it was good to stretch her legs and get a breath of fresh air. Ms. Murphy thought she could walk farther but worried she would not have enough energy to make the grueling climb back up to her apartment. Unable to lift herself using only her legs, Ms. Murphy pulled herself up the stairs, white knuckles gripping the wooden bannister with fierce determination. The one flight of stairs took her more than five minutes to climb, pausing every few steps to catch her breath. Still, Ms. Murphy thought the chance to observe the goings-on of the church, feel the air, and take part in the life of the city were worth the treacherous climb.

Ms. Murphy was just beginning to come to terms with the idea that her health was unlikely to improve. A little more than a year before we met, she had traveled to London and Ireland to visit her family. At the time, she did not realize that it was likely her last visit home. Only in her late sixties, she was relatively young to be experiencing such significant debility. The accumulated years—many of struggle and poverty—had taken their toll.

Ms. Murphy was born in rural County Cork, Ireland, in the thin years between the World Wars. Her unmarried mother worked as a live-in maid and was unable to keep her job and care for an infant, so Ms. Murphy became a ward of the state before she could walk. Fostered as the eldest girl in a large farm family, she left high school before graduating. She was needed on the farm. The land was too poor to provide even for her foster family, so Ms. Murphy learned as a teenager that she and most of her foster siblings would have to seek a living elsewhere. She decided nursing would suit her better than teaching; these were the only two middle-class occupations available to young women at the time. Jobs in Ireland were scarce in those days, so Ms. Murphy applied to nursing schools in London. She finished her high school courses at night after long days of nursing training. When she finished training, she worked for a few years in English hospitals. Seeking relief from ongoing postwar rations, she applied to hospitals across the former British colonies before finally deciding to accept an offer from a Jewish hospital on Chicago's north side. Ms. Murphy arrived in Chicago knowing no one, but she quickly acquired lifelong friends—other nurses, her landlord's family, distant relatives, and other Irish immigrants. Her early years in Chicago were good ones: her face lit up with remembered excitement when she spoke about dancing in the ballrooms of the era. Those carefree days ended when her friends married and had children. She remained single and never once mentioned to me if she had ever hoped for such a family herself.

Ms. Murphy worked at the same hospital for 30 years, mostly on the floor they called Hollywood, a floor nobody wanted. It was the ward for children with terminal cases. She worked nights, often the only nurse on the shift. She became an expert on cancer, tuberculosis, and late-stage diabetes. Late-stage everything, really. Alone with dying children and frantic mothers in the small hours, Ms. Murphy learned to listen; she learned to hear what her patients really needed. She learned to care. She recalled difficult conversations with terminal patients: "'Nurse,' they'd say, 'I'm only going to be here a short time. I'm going to the great beyond.'" Ms. Murphy learned to think fast, the only thing to say: "We're all going to go there eventually; we'll meet you there." "Good," she recalled one patient responding, "so you'll take care of me up there too?" After she stopped working on Hollywood, Ms. Murphy worked as a supervising nurse in a nursing home, and then for an expensive private-duty home care company whose patients required round-the-clock care. Before she needed care herself, Ms. Murphy had spent her life caring for the sick, the frail, the terminally ill.

Ms. Murphy came to rely on her expansive web of friends as she became more frail, her rheumatoid arthritis swelling and stiffening her joints. One friend brought her groceries and picked up her prescriptions. Another drove her to the bank. A third, the daughter of a friend, took her for her haircuts every six weeks. But as her friends experienced health crises of their own or moved nearer to children, Ms. Murphy quickly found herself struggling to keep fresh food and medicine in the house.

By the time we met, Ms. Murphy was an old hand at starting life afresh, at making the best of things, and at caring. Unlike many older adults, Ms. Murphy did not wait until a hospitalization forced her to get some help at home. She knew the path ahead and knew what services were available to help her. First, she tried to get government-subsidized care through the CCP, but at the time her retirement savings were too substantial to qualify. So, she hired Belltower, a local agency that had a good reputation. She could only afford about eight hours of help a week. She hoped that would be enough. Belltower sent Sally to be her home care worker. Sally helped Ms. Murphy with her laundry, cooking, and cleaning. She monitored Ms. Murphy's showers, making sure the older woman did not slip and fall. Sally did not drive, and so I was soon running errands, grocery shopping, and picking up prescriptions for Ms. Murphy, drawn into the fragile web of care that she kept reconstructing around her.

Not quite a year after I met Ms. Murphy, she spent a week in the hospital recovering from a bout of vomiting that had left her weakened and with precariously low blood pressure. She went into the hospital on a Tuesday, and though many of her friends called, I was the only person able to visit her until the following weekend. Her carefully nurtured web of friends could not sustain her any longer. After Ms. Murphy was released from the hospital, Sally stayed with her around the clock, sleeping on Ms. Murphy's couch, which looked like it was purchased some time in the 1960s. Frustrated and tired, Sally soon decided to retire from home care altogether.[15]

Putting on a brave face, Ms. Murphy tried to adjust to her new home care worker, Irene Cruz. Belltower supervisors tried to patch the tattered web of support that enabled Ms. Murphy to live at home by coordinating with Meals-on-Wheels to bring her prepared meals. By the time Ms. Murphy and I sat down to record her life history, we both saw the writing on the wall: She would not remain at home much longer. Reminiscing about her childhood on the farm, about her long years as a nurse, Ms. Murphy connected impending changes to those in her past. When she spoke of elder care, she spoke not only as a person receiving care, but also as someone who had spent her life caring for vulnerable and dying people.

Sally had given her good care—Ms. Murphy knew because "I was a nurse, that's why. I have a good idea what's good care and what's not." The key to caring for someone well was to get to know them really know them. And the only way to know a person was to talk to them and really listen to what they say. By encouraging patients to talk about themselves, she learned "what their biggest problem was. Was it the fact that they couldn't go out and take care of themselves? Or was it the fact they didn't like so many people around them all the time? You had to go different ways to see what they want. Some of them would say, 'I don't like those damn nurses. They're all over the place.' Then I would know it was time to slow it down a bit." For Ms. Murphy, listening to patients was not only about gathering diagnostically useful information about a patient's bodily ailments. Listening also helped her learn which social arrangements of care worked best for each patient. Ms. Murphy imagined care as extending beyond attention to physical ailments; care also meant attuning the social relations of care to each patient's subjectivity. This might mean enabling a patient to be more self-sufficient, minimizing the number of people around, or slowing down the pace of activity. She expected similar attunements from those who now cared for her.

Unlike Sally, who was brisk, quiet, and unemotional, Irene fussed over Ms. Murphy. She described Irene as "a little on the motherly type. I never had that kind of stuff, you know. I was always much more to myself. Kids in Ireland in those days they didn't get a lot of fuss made out of them. Especially if you were in a farming community like I was because they were all so busy." Ms. Murphy speculated that perhaps Irene's more intrusive style of care and direct manner of asking questions were encouraged in Irene's native Philippines. While many older adults might have appreciated Irene's warmth, Ms. Murphy interpreted Irene's attentions as a kind of motherly coddling—they made her feel like she was a brainless person or a child, instead of a competent adult in need of assistance. Sally's more distant, formal manner and her proficiency with household tasks meant that she was able to care for Ms. Murphy in a manner that reproduced social relations of care similar to those in Ms. Murphy's youth.

At stake in care for Ms. Murphy was the familiarity of social relations and the ways in which relations with care workers might sustain or threaten her inclusion in human social worlds. She evaluated care based on "how they treat me. I want them to treat me like I'm a human being, and I have a few brains left too. I don't like when they treat me like I'm an imbecile, like I'm upset. At first, Irene would ask me about my medication: 'Why are you taking it? Why do you have arthritis?' I don't know. It just came. I didn't go around looking for it." The tone of Irene's questions put Ms. Murphy on the defensive. She resented the implication that she was somehow responsible for her own suffering and did not understand her own bodily condition. Irene implied that Ms. Murphy's inability to answer such questions was a sign of cognitive decline. Ms. Murphy saw that same inability as a sign of her humility in the face of the unknowable. The question of why she had arthritis was a religious one for Ms. Murphy—who was she to know God's reasons? Ms. Murphy wanted to be recognized for her continued ability to make sense in and of a complex world, as opposed to being cared for in a way that sought evidence of her limitations.

When I asked Ms. Murphy what she sought in care, she told me, "If I have my senses at all, I'd like to be treated like I have some. I'd like to be treated as a person, not a piece of furniture." Ms. Murphy used the phrase "having my senses" expansively. It meant more than cognitive competence, but also her sensibilities. If those who cared for her failed to recognize that she had "a few brains left," they might also fail to treat her as human at all.[16] Such care might hasten social death,[17] treating her as an object, a piece of furniture, something to be dusted or plumped or rearranged around a room but never asked for an opinion. Good care, then, was not simply care that enabled Ms. Murphy to live at home, or care that sustained her health. Good care also needed to recognize and sustain her personhood.

Home care workers' technical proficiency in tasks like cleaning and cooking were thus prerequisite to, but not sufficient for, good care. Such tasks could only sustain personhood when they were attuned to elders' lifetimes of embodied experience. For Ms. Murphy, care was not about independence as a rigid moral good, but about recognizing individuals' personhood by sustaining their ways of life. The responsive adaptations that Sally made—her unfussy demeanor, her attention to cooking Ms. Murphy's favorite Irish dishes according to the older woman's preferences, making time to take walks with her—incorporated the older woman's subjectivity into everyday care practices. Sally attuned her care to Ms. Murphy's lifetimes of experience, habits, preferences, and relationships and thereby treated her as a valued participant in social life: a person.

It's according to the Person

"If the Lord said to me, 'Hattie, you can have one thing,' it would be a daughter. If I could have one thing in this world, it would be a daughter." Hattie Meyers's deep voice bore the warm sound of her upbringing in small-town Alabama. Her easy laughter belied her ongoing grief over the deaths of her husband and both her sons many years earlier. Mrs. Meyers was a survivor, though she was not quite sure how she had managed to live so much longer than her kin. Speaking of their deaths, she told me, "I lived through it. I made it somehow." Mrs. Meyers had been making it through, somehow, for more than 80 years by the time we met, and very little of her life had been easy. The road from a childhood shaped by the violence of being black in the Jim Crow South to a more prosperous, politically connected, middle-class adulthood in Chicago had indelibly shaped Mrs. Meyers's worldview. These experiences left her deeply empathetic toward the struggles of her home care workers and simultaneously distrustful of them.

For all her losses, Mrs. Meyers carried herself with the demeanor of a matriarch. With no kin living nearby, she gathered friends and neighbors close. There was Rock, who lived upstairs and checked in on her several times a day. It was Rock who called 911 when Mrs. Meyers had a severe diabetic episode. Afterward, it was Rock who made sure the medical supply company delivered everything she needed to come home. Mandy lived downstairs. When Mandy moved into the building ten years earlier with her young son, Mrs. Meyers worried about her because "she just didn't know anything." Mrs. Meyers took Mandy under her wing, inviting the young mother to Christmas dinner when she realized Mandy planned to serve sandwiches. In the years since, Mandy had become the daughter Mrs. Meyers never had, calling the older woman "Ma." Mandy drove Mrs. Meyers to the store and to doctors' appointments.

Even though Mrs. Meyers longed for daughterly relationships, she objected when her home care worker Loretta Gordon called her "Ma." She worried Loretta might take advantage of any motherly affection she developed. It had happened before with other workers. Sometimes Loretta complained that Mrs. Meyers was so suspicious of her. Loretta insisted she had never done anything to earn such distrust. Mrs. Meyers learned early on that even the most respected people could let you down, be selfish, and cause harm. If family was not exempt from causing pain, neither was anyone else.

Mrs. Meyers's understanding of what it meant to be a person had been deeply shaped by long experience of pain and hardship. Some of these experiences were directly related to the racism she encountered as a young child in Alabama and as an adult in Chicago. Others were the indirect result of living in a world in which health and health care are unevenly distributed by race and class. Mrs. Meyers was less explicitly interested in independence than some older adults. Instead, Mrs. Meyers had a deeply relational sense of personhood. Who a person was, she implied, depended on their experiences. Good care had to be based on each person's idiosyncrasies—on their history and how it shaped what they wanted in life. She knew from her own experiences in domestic work and her long history with care workers that many faced serious hardships. Her distrust of Loretta did not imply judgment. It reflected Mrs. Meyers's recognition of a familiar, painful history.

Born in the parsonage of a small town in rural Alabama, Mrs. Meyers was raised by her maternal grandmother. Her mother died in childbirth when Mrs. Meyers was one year old. Her grandmother blamed her father for her mother's death, believing that he had been an inadequate breadwinner. Mrs. Meyers described her father, the only child of a deaf and mute woman who had never been able to work, as someone who had "raised himself, went to school and taught himself, went to the army." When Mrs. Meyers was young, her father was the only black brick mason in town, and the only black bondsman. She spoke proudly of the respect he garnered in their town: "He was a smart man. He would go to work in the morning. He never missed a day. He always had good ideas. He had to. You could see him standing on the street in the morning and all these white guys with their suits and ties on go ahead and getting ready to go to their businesses talking to my father. He had money in the bank, but it wasn't much. He wasn't known as a dummy, but he didn't give us a lot."

When Mrs. Meyers's mother died, her grandmother first assumed responsibility for her and her three siblings. For all his success, Mrs. Meyers's father did not give his children or their grandmother money to support them. Her grandmother, a laundress whose husband worked at the cotton mill, could not afford to care for all four children. Eventually, Mrs. Meyers's siblings were sent to live with other kin. Throughout their childhood, her siblings begged to come back to live with their grandmother. Mrs. Meyers attributed many of her siblings' problems later in life to the difficulties they faced in other households.

Mrs. Meyers's elder sister Milly had it the hardest. She lived with their father and his mother. Milly suffered from what Mrs. Meyers called "sleeping sickness" and did poorly in school. Their father made Milly leave school to work as a maid when she was barely a teenager. The consequences of this work weighed heavily on Mrs. Meyers, who remembered how Milly was "really pretty, but was bounced around from this lady to that . . . My father would send her or let her go with anybody. My sister went to work real young. I just want to tell you this one thing, because it's always on my mind and has made me do a lot that I didn't expect." Mrs. Meyers paused and took a deep breath before continuing, "When I was real small and Milly was only 13 or so—she worked for some people that had her taking care of this older white man. I remember one Saturday evening, she used to hate so bad to go up there, these people would go off and she'd go take care, and she took me with her, and he was a mean old man, hollering and saying dirty things and calling us names. Racist names." The names were bad enough. But as Mrs.

Meyers continued her story, she told me that Milly was also sexually abused by the older man and by at least one other employer.

Mrs. Meyers also experienced the sexual perils of domestic work. Starting at the age of 15, she worked before and after school as a maid for the Carpenter family. Her sister-in-law Arlene worked for them too, and got her the job. She started working for them full time after she graduated from high school. She remembered the lady of the house as "such a sweet lady" who owned a boutique and had beautiful clothes. Mrs. Carpenter was generous with her employees. Her husband was another story. Mrs. Meyers recalled, "My sister-in-law was going with Mr. Carpenter. All the black women in town, he sold cars and you'd pass by there and he was winking at you . . . He would come back home after Mrs. Carpenter went to work. They had a closed-in back porch, and he would go in there and take off all his clothes, and you'd see him walking around the kitchen buck naked." Mrs. Meyers raised her eyebrows, looking to see if I understood her horror at this. She continued, telling me that she told Mr. Carpenter, "Now you better get out of here because my name is not Arlene and I don't go with white men." Her refusals did not stop him from repeated harassment. She said, "He did that for so long. But I was old enough, and smart enough to know that I got to do something to not take this anymore."

One day, Mrs. Carpenter chastised her for not having the kitchen cleaned up from breakfast when she and her husband came home for lunch. She responded that she had not had time because of other chores. Her rebuttal angered Mr. Carpenter, who, she remembered, said, "Let me tell you one damn thing. I don't allow no black bitches to talk to my wife like that." That was the last straw for Mrs. Meyers, who knew that he was angry that she had refused his advances. She recalled, "I was at the point in my life where I don't feel like I should take that, and it made me so angry. I love Mrs. Carpenter so much, so I hated to hurt her. I really believed she knew that he was trying to go with all black women. I started telling him off and I couldn't stop. I knew better but I couldn't stop. I was so mad at him because what had gotten into me was 'I ain't going to take it no more. You just not going to do me like this.' I called him a so-and-so peckerwood. I left then and went home. Went and told my daddy." Mrs. Meyers paused, her eyes registering the fear she felt when her father confronted Mr. Carpenter: "Daddy went up there and told him don't bother with her. I left right after that. Daddy sent me to St. Louis where my sister lived. My dad was proud of me because I tried to conduct myself well. He was very angry too, because for him to go and talk to that white guy, he had to be angry. They could always have hung him for it. I could have come to St. Louis before then, but I didn't, I didn't want to leave my grandmother."

Mrs. Meyers and her sisters' experiences were common across the South, where black domestic workers were particularly vulnerable to employers' sexual assaults. Historian Marcia Chatelain notes that many families sent young girls North to protect them from entry into "the labor market at a young age and from the sexual vulnerability and constant threats to their personal safety due to racist practices of their bosses, and little protection from the police or courts."[18] Sending daughters northward also protected male relatives who felt duty bound to protect their kinswomen, but faced severe violence and economic reprisals for so doing.

Aware that sexual assault against domestic workers was widespread, Mrs. Meyers attributed her escape from such assault to the relatively later age at which she went into service and to the confidence instilled by her grandmother. She contrasted her resistance to Mr. Carpenter's advances to her sister Milly's inability to ward off similar abuse. Left without their grandmother's protection, and "slow" in school, Milly had been sent to work very young. Mrs. Meyers felt ongoing regret and guilt over her sister's hardships. She worried constantly about Milly, who even in her late eighties was living in a house Mrs. Meyers described as "totally drug infested." Mrs. Meyers blamed Milly's lifelong struggles on the exploitation, violence, and trauma she experienced as a young domestic worker. Mrs. Meyers saw Milly in the faces of the many exhausted home care workers she had met over the years, some of whom also lived with abuse and addiction. She knew intimately the dangers of work that occurred behind closed doors. Mrs. Meyers never explicitly linked her and her sister's experiences with those of her home care workers. Yet when Mrs. Meyers spoke about the home care workers she thought were untrustworthy, she always explained that they were "in trouble." She blamed their faults as care workers on their circumstances rather than their characters. I heard echoes of her compassion for her sister in her compassion for home care workers, and echoes of her frustration with her sister's perpetual crises in her frustration with workers' personal problems.

After leaving Alabama, Mrs. Meyers got a job in St. Louis working in a glass factory, and met her husband soon after. She liked him because he was a working man, a butcher with a steady job at one of the meatpacking houses. He seemed like he would be a good family man—unlike her father, he was someone she thought she could really rely on. They had two sons. When Mr. Meyers's St. Louis packing plant closed down, he found a job at another one in Chicago, and they moved north. Around the time their boys started school, the packing plant in Chicago also closed, forcing Mr. Meyers to take a lower paying job. Mrs. Meyers returned to work. She held a string of clerical jobs for Cook County, and got involved in local Democratic party politics. She eventually used those political connections to get a job as county Deputy Sheriff. These were good years for Mrs. Meyers. There was enough money, and her boys were still healthy. She was even able to do a little traveling and go to the theater. It was a far cry from her childhood, scrubbing laundry in Alabama. She recalled, "Outside of work, I had a lot of friends. We had a club, like we went to Las Vegas two or three times a year. We went to Hawaii, we went on a couple of cruises. We had a club and we'd take up money, we'd always be going downtown to some kind of show. We did a lot of things at that time."

Upward mobility did not insulate Mrs. Meyers from the racism and troubles of the time. She spoke frequently of the horror she felt during the 1968 Chicago riots when she was tasked as a Sheriff's Deputy with driving executives to their suburban homes from their offices downtown. Forty years later, her voice cracked with pain and fury as she remembered feeling impotent as she drove them through her own burning West-side neighborhood. Her fury was the weary kind, the kind so accustomed to an unjust world that she recalled not being the least bit surprised that law enforcement spent more resources on chauffeuring rich white men than protecting the homes and livelihoods of black families.

Though Mrs. Meyers and her husband had made good incomes when they were working, they were never able to save much. They once owned a nice house in a good neighborhood on Chicago's west side, but redlining, white flight, and mounting violence depleted its value by the time Mrs. Meyers sold it several decades later. The symptoms of her husband's multiple sclerosis (MS) had accumulated gradually. When he could no longer work, he started drinking heavily. Mrs. Meyers cared for her husband at home for years with the help of her sons. His drinking made him suicidal and abusive. When it got too bad, Mrs. Meyers decided she could no longer care for him at home. She sold their house and moved herself and her sons to a two-bedroom apartment in the same neighborhood. Her husband moved into a nursing home, where she visited daily. He told her that a "man had beat him up, a guy that worked there. I didn't know what to do. I was afraid that if I'd tell somebody they'd beat him up [again]." The experience made her wary of trusting the care of her kin to strangers.

Mrs. Meyers's distrust of caregivers grew when her son Tommy started needing care; he also had MS. Tommy was in college and working nights when he started having problems with his vision—he lost his sight completely within a year. Tommy lived in supportive housing for several years, but Mrs. Meyers eventually brought him home. She hired home care workers to help him when she was at work. It was an infuriating experience. She told me, "All kinds of stuff they stole from me. So I got rid of the one and got someone else. One evening, I had opened the door and came in and she had a great big pot on the stove and it was boiling and she was laying there asleep. Tommy was in there calling her. That broke my heart. That pot was just boiling over. I got rid of her. Just one thing after another." She continued, "Tommy got worse and worse. So eventually I retired. I returned and came home and took care of him myself; it was hard. He needed help for eight years, and my husband needed help for about twenty." She remembered, "All this time, I also had to go see about my husband because he was getting worse. When he died, Tommy had gotten into such a bad condition he wasn't able to go to his father's funeral or anything. Everything died in his body and he was such a good and intelligent young man. I was strong and determined to take care of my husband and my son. I got through it. It broke me down so much." Unable to find trustworthy care workers, Mrs. Meyers retired to care for her son herself. In the process, she lost the social connections and the income her job provided. The effort had taken an emotional, physical, and financial toll.

In Mrs. Meyers's telling, the deaths of her husband and son, only a few years apart, had the strange quality of being both expected and shocking. Even deaths that come slowly surprise in their finality. Only five years after Tommy died, Mrs. Meyers's eldest son Brandon died of complications related to diabetes. Mrs. Meyers had not quite made sense of this last and most unexpected death. Brandon had lived with her most of his life, helping care for Tommy when he wasn't working as a machinist at a candy factory. Bewilderment and devastation lingered in her telling of his passing. She took long gulping pauses as she spoke, as if summoning up the stamina to put into words what she still could not understand: "We didn't even know Brandon had sugar [diabetes] until . . . Brandon was real quiet . . . If I had known his feet was like it was. He had gangrene all over his . . . When he got in that hospital, they had his foot . . . he wasn't even there an hour before they had his foot off. Three days, they had cut him three times, his knees and above his knees. But anyways, I lived through it . . . Once Brandon went into the hospital, he never came out." Mrs. Meyers explained that Brandon had never complained about pain in his foot, and they had no idea he was diabetic: "He wouldn't tell. He thought because his father and his brother had been so sick, he just didn't want to worry me." Mrs. Meyers could never quite tell me how many years it had been since Brandon's death. More than a decade, certainly. His bedroom remained much as he had left it, decorated with musical instruments and concert posters, reminders of a vibrant young man. Mrs. Meyers did not hide the toll these hardships had taken, readily expressing her ongoing pain. She carried the weight of this history as part of her buoyant, clear-eyed tenacity.

Long a caregiver to her kin, Mrs. Meyers was left without nearby kin to look after her in her old age. For a long time, she stitched together support from the neighbors she gathered to her. Eventually she needed more regular help than they could provide. Her diabetes, asthma, and other health problems were difficult to manage. Though Mrs. Meyers's family had once been comfortably middle-class, medical expenses eventually ate away at their savings. By the time Mrs. Meyers needed care, her assets were depleted and she qualified for publicly funded care from Plusmore. During one of her frequent hospitalizations several years before we met, a social worker had finally managed to convince Mrs. Meyers that she needed help at home. Distrustful and guarded, she eventually agreed.

Mrs. Meyers made sense of paid care through these earlier experiences of racial and gendered violence. She did not want to be taken advantage of. If possible, she wanted to be cared for by those who would honestly keep track of what they were supposed to do without her constantly having to remind them. She understood that the women who cared for her often lived troubled lives. She saw in them the echoes of her past. They were constant reminders of who she might have been but for a few small accidents of history.

Mrs. Meyers had been through dozens of home care workers. Loretta had been working with her for nearly a year. Mrs. Meyers spoke of Loretta as hardworking and secretive: "She'll mop and wax my bedroom floor. None of them others did that. She'll do it if I tell her. She'll put my curtains up. She'll make my cornbread and okra. They won't do it. She's just as sweet as a button if you're looking right at her face, but it's not really who she is. You have to know that she's hiding something." Mrs. Meyers continued her simultaneously critical and compassionate evaluation of Loretta, "She's not mean to me or anything. She would never be mean to me. She's just in a lot of trouble but she will try to make you think that she is not. . . . She forget and burn your bread or lose something or move your pocketbook so you can't find it, but she's got kind of that fault, but there's a lot of good things about Loretta. She has been here longer than any of them."

It mattered to Mrs. Meyers that workers stayed around. So many left when they found jobs that were better paying or offered more hours. She asked to have some of them replaced because they showed up sick, or drunk, or refused to do the work the company assigned them. It was always a disaster when she had to replace a worker. Sometimes Plusmore had to send three or four (and one time nearly a dozen) workers before they sent someone Mrs. Meyers thought was adequate. It was scary and unsettling to have so many strangers in her home, so Mrs. Meyers had learned to make do with "good enough" workers like Loretta rather than hoping for someone who was a perfect fit.

Despite Mrs. Meyers's compassion for Loretta, she wished she could find a worker who would figure out what to do without much instruction or supervision. For Mrs. Meyers, this was critical—she wanted care from someone she did not have to monitor. She wanted care that did not have to be announced or supervised. She did not like being in the position of an employer, she did not like managing her care workers as the white women of her youth had once managed her. When I asked her outright what she thought made good care, or what it meant to take good care of someone, she told me, "I'm not sure, because it's according to who you're taking care of and according to what they want. I'm not that easy to take care of, I guess. I'd like for someone to come in and do what they supposed to." Mrs. Meyers continued, "Like I told Loretta when she came in here. 'Look, Loretta, you just do what you know you're supposed to do and that is just good. I don't want to have to tell you because I may want you to wash on Monday and you don't feel like washing on Monday. Maybe you'd rather wash on Wednesday. Just so you wash that week.' But she'll wait a month. I just wear a lot of stuff and I said, 'I got to have something to wear around in the house.' She said 'Yeah, okay, Ma. I'll go wash.' She'll go wash right then but I got to remind her. . . . I'd like them to come in and do what they know that they should do without me having to worry about: I need the wash, I need her to do this, I need her to do that."

Like both Ms. Murphy and Mrs. Cole, Mrs. Meyers saw care as inherently responsive to the subjectivities of those cared for, as responsive to the person. Many older adults shared these women's desire for workers who did not require instruction. They preferred workers who could work in the style often described to me as "independently." Care workers who worked "independently" supported older adults' sense of independence. For many older adults, constantly describing each detail of how they liked their home kept or meals cooked meant repeatedly announcing their vulnerability and lack of self-sufficiency. Like Mrs. Meyers, nearly every older adult I spoke to in Chicago told me that one crucial component of "good care" was that the worker "just knew" what needed to be done in their home.

Mrs. Meyers's vision of good care was deeply situational. Her ideal form of care depended on the desires of those being cared for, but could flexibly accommodate care workers' circumstances. She was all too familiar with the kinds of hardship that women in domestic service faced and tried to be compassionate about their limitations. Mrs. Meyers felt ambivalent about her relationships with care workers. Unlike Mrs. Cole, she preferred not to think of them as employees whom she could boss around. But she was also wary of thinking of workers as kin, since she was anxious that they might take advantage of the reciprocities implied by such relations.

In telling her life story, Mrs. Meyers had little to say about being or becoming independent. Rather, she spoke of the ways that care, concern, and money had circulated among kin, protecting some and paving the path to violence for others. She saw clearly the ways that care given or withheld could shape personhood, marking the difference between her relatively stability and her sister's ongoing insecurity.

Generating Persons

The ways that people morally imagine both their own personhood and that of others are culturally and historically contingent, but also reflect their particular histories of experience. Older adults' life histories highlight the multiplicity of ways in which people come to understand the concepts of personhood and independence. These older adults shared broad, normative Euro-American cultural interests in sustaining liberal personhood through care. Yet their understandings of personhood were also generated through experiences of care, kinship, success, loss, and violence. These experiences, in turn, reflected their different racial, economic, and geographic locations and were marked by their different engagements in broad historical processes and shifts.

Despite this diversity, older Chicagoans shared a sense that care should continue to sustain them as individual persons with subjectivities that reflected their distinct experiences. They believed that good care was care that was attuned to their unique, individual person and continued to sustain them as this kind of person. Achieving this kind of care required workers to have immense empathic capacity and a willingness to sustain the personhood of others, even when doing so threatened their own well-being. Much as older adults' understandings of personhood develop through lifetimes of experience, workers' ethics of care reflected their diverse life histories. It is to workers' life histories of care, violence, and survival that I now turn.

2

Inheriting Care

Home Care Workers' Lives

Doris Robinson's eyebrow lifted in an expression I had come to recognize as bemused patience. I was helping her dust her elderly client's bedroom. Our conversation veered towards her concerns about her grandson, Teshawn, who lived with her. He had been born two months early, and she was concerned that at a year old he had yet to roll over. Eager to be useful, I began offering Doris advice about how to access public services that could test Teshawn for developmental disabilities and link him to interventions. When I finished my soliloquy, Doris gently let me know that she had already made an appointment for him to be assessed. Her own dyslexia had remained undiagnosed until ninth grade. Doris was not about to let her grandson fall through the same cracks. Those forced to navigate the punitive and labyrinthine US social welfare system develop substantial bureaucratic expertise.

Doris's bemusement was justified—she was a veteran of fragmented social service systems across three states. Doris knew exactly what time to start standing in line when she needed to talk to someone at the Social Security office about the disability insurance she received because of her lupus. She knew whom to call to avoid getting the run-around if there was a problem with her Medicaid benefits. This hard-won expertise made it possible for her and her family to survive even though she could only work part time and earned something like $8.90 an hour.

As is true for many home care workers, much of what made Doris an excellent home care worker had been learned in the process of caring for herself and her family. Doris's home care client, John Thomas, once worked in the finance department of a major candy company. He had substantial savings and a pension. He did not need to rely on public programs for health or home care. Doris still put her bureaucratic skills to use on his behalf. Once, I listened as Doris wheedled the optometrist's receptionist to make an appointment for Mr. Thomas during the doctor's regular lunch hour, arguing that it was the only time that Mr. Thomas would have the energy for such a trip when Doris would be available to accompany him.

The life stories of home care workers expose the way that women's generative labor links care, kinship, labor, and poverty. For many care workers, as anthropologist Leith Mullings observes is true for many African American women, "building a family is inherently an act of resistance" against an ongoing racial order that persistently threatens and devalues people of color.[1] Before taking home care jobs, many workers develop necessary expertise while caring for kin amid scarcity and violence. At an early age, many learn to navigate low-wage jobs and the maze of social services to acquire the necessities of daily life while protecting the integrity of their families. As workers learn to care with kin, they also develop forms of moral imagination in which care practices are embedded in broader kinship practices characterized by obligation, reciprocity, and sacrifice. Home care agencies put both their expertise and their moral imaginations to work, turning those qualities into something that can be bought and sold at an hourly rate. Yet home care agencies, funded by limited government reimbursements or by elders' often-limited budgets, cannot afford to pay workers living wages. Home care workers continue to live in poverty, despite their generative labor that makes possible the lives of both kin and clients.

In what follows, I review the seemingly separate histories of US labor law, elder care policy, and anti-poverty programs to show the role of these programs in creating a home care workforce comprised primarily of women from low-income families of color. These broader histories form the invisible foundation upon which home care workers' lives play out, shaping the possibilities and challenges that workers navigate as they try to make life possible for themselves and their kin. I then turn to workers' life histories, which illustrate how workers draw creatively from their experiences with kin to care for clients. They adapt familial habits to care for older adults while simultaneously struggling to care for their own families. Workers' life histories show how the social, familial, and institutional contexts in which these women became workers continue to shape their everyday care practices and ethical commitments to care.[2] These histories also provide intimate accounts of the ways that poverty and inequality are interwoven with care. Many discussions of poor women of color in the United States focus on the reproduction of poverty in their lives. Home care workers' stories also foreground their profound creativity in the face of racism and hardship, and their crucial role generating the independence of others within the inescapable interdependencies that make human life possible.

National Inheritance as Familial Inheritance

Contemporary home care workers' lives are shaped by social and policy legacies engendering domestic work and caregiving in the United States. Home care workers cared for kin and clients in the midst of intergenerational poverty. Their poverty was the consequence of long histories of racial and ethnic discrimination perpetuated by the low wages they earn as care workers. Throughout the history of the country, it has been common for poor women and women of color to generate the lives of wealthier households. These legacies leave women of color stretched thin, struggling to provide both the care required by their employers and the care needed by their own families. The current concentration of women and families of color in low-wage domestic and care work is a legacy perpetuated by discriminatory laws and policies. It is in this sense that black feminist theorists Maxine Baca Zinn and Bonnie Thornton Dill argue that "labor relations are at the core of race and gender inequalities."[3] Workers' different life histories must be understood within the context of this broader sociopolitical inheritance.

Prior to the development of the public welfare state in the mid-twentieth century, most care for those considered dependent—children, people with disabilities, and the elderly—was provided within families and communities.[4] Then, as now, race and class played a substantial role in determining how care was provided. Little care was available to indigent older white adults without kin, who were relegated to institutions called "poorhouses" or "almshouses" where charities and local governments provided food and shelter. The able-bodied were required to work to offset costs. Almshouses offered minimal health care to the chronically ill. Enslaved black Americans depended on other slaves for care as they aged. Some have argued that favored domestic slaves were well cared for by slave owners in old age; however, the historical record suggests that owners regularly neglected slaves who were unable to work. After abolition, most institutions caring for the aged remained racially segregated.[5]

Intimacy and exploitation have long been intricately connected in domestic work in the United States, challenging widespread assumptions that domestic spaces are spaces of safety, affection, and mutuality.[6] In most communities of the late eighteenth and early nineteenth centuries, women were primarily responsible for the care of kin, though wealthier women could employ domestic servants to do the bulk of the bodily labor involved in such care. During this era in the northern and western United States, immigrant women from Southern Europe, Asia, and Latin America filled these positions along with young white women from poor families.[7] Prior to abolition, in the US South, black slave women provided much of the care and domestic service required by wealthier white older adults. After abolition, violence and discrimination continued to restrict employment opportunities, pushing many women of color into domestic and agricultural work.

Between 1910 and 1970, approximately six million black American women and men joined the Great Migration to northern cities, fleeing violence and discrimination in the Jim Crow South.[8] Employment restrictions in the North also limited the opportunities available to black men and women. Discrimination depressed black men's wages, such that few earned enough to support families according to the era's ideal of the male-breadwinner, female-homemaker model of domestic life. Black women were thus more likely to participate in the paid workforce than their white counterparts. Facing discrimination that kept them out of better paying jobs in northern cities, many black women entered domestic service. There, at least, domestic workers were more likely to successfully refuse live-in employment than had been possible in the South.

The Great Depression provided the impetus for the first federally funded caregiving programs in the United States. Between 1929 and 1939, widespread unemployment and poverty devastated families across the country, leaving them struggling to care for elderly kin. Desperate families increasingly left older adults at public hospitals, which soon filled to capacity. The Works Progress Administration (WPA), a New Deal recovery program implemented in 1935 to provide public jobs to families, developed the first federally funded paid caregiving services.[9] Fearing that direct income supports would breed dependence, New Deal reformers billed the WPA jobs initiatives as an anti-poverty measure that would instill independence through labor.[10] Alongside the WPA's more famous large construction projects which created jobs for men, the administration created several smaller programs, like the Housekeeping Service for Chronic Patients, which employed visiting housekeeping aides to care for children and people with chronic illnesses. The Housekeeping Service achieved dual goals by relieving public hospitals of the burden of chronic care and employing poor women.

The Housekeeping Service reproduced existing hierarchies of gender, race, and class. The WPA only funded one job per household, which typically went to men in married couples. For this reason, most of the Housekeeping Service's employees were divorcees and widows. Advocates successfully pushed for the WPA to pay white female heads of household to care for their own children. Black women were denied these benefits, pushing them into Housekeeping Service jobs. This policy officially devalued the work black (but not white) women did to sustain their families and subsidized racial discrimination.[11] As a result, four out of five aides employed by the Housekeeping Service 1938 were black American women.

The Fair Labor Standards Act (FLSA), another piece of New Deal legislation passed in 1938, further entrenched the era's racialized class hierarchies. The FLSA set a federal minimum wage, guaranteed overtime pay, and outlawed child labor in most occupations. The bill threatened to upend the racial caste system upon which the economies of former slave states depended. A legislative compromise necessary to pass the FLSA excluded domestic and agricultural workers from FLSA protections. As a result of discriminatory hiring, both occupational sectors were disproportionately filled by workers of color. The FLSA thereby codified pre–Civil War racial divisions of labor for the remainder of the twentieth century. Excluding agricultural and domestic workers from FLSA's protections ensured the continued low wages and enhanced the profitability of these industries at the expense of poor workers of color.[12]

In 1974, the US Congress amended the FLSA, finally extending its protections to most domestic workers. It continued to exclude two kinds of employees: "casual" babysitters and those providing "companionship" services to individuals unable to care for themselves due to age or infirmity.[13] The companionship exemption was interpreted as excluding paid home care workers from the FLSA's protections.[14] The Department of Labor issued new rules in 2013 that interpreted the FLSA as including home care workers. After protracted legal battles, the new rules went into effect in 2016, finally extending minimum wage and overtime protections to home care workers.[15]

In addition to work programs and labor protections, the New Deal created several programs to assist older adults. By the 1930s, older adults formed the largest group of people in poverty. The United States had changed from a primarily agricultural economy to an industrial one. This made the practice of older adults continuing to work into late life and then be cared for in homes by kin increasingly untenable. Older workers had a hard time finding jobs in the new economy. The Social Security insurance program, passed in 1935, sought to provide older adults the means to retire by providing those over the age of 65 with a monthly income.[16] Though Social Security provided older adults with income support, these benefits were inadequate to fund rising medical costs.

By 1965, nearly one out of three older adults did not have health insurance, and many could not afford the out-of-pocket costs of medical care. That year, the federal government created the Medicare and Medicaid programs, fundamentally changing the way that the United States provides care to older adults. In an era when the duration, intensity, and expense of caring for older adults expanded dramatically, Medicare and Medicaid alleviated pressure on families by shifting some costs to state and federal governments. Medicare also required hospitals and doctors' offices to become racially integrated in order to receive funding, radically expanding health care access for millions of Americans.[17]

Programs targeting care for older adults are typically considered distinct from programs targeting poor children and families. Yet aging policy and anti-poverty policies have complex, tangled effects on the lives of multigenerational families and the families of care workers. From 1935 until the mid-1990s, the nation's largest anti-poverty program, Aid to Dependent Children (ADC, later known as Aid to Families with Dependent Children, or AFDC) provided cash benefits to poor single mothers raising minor children, enabling them to care for their children without entering the workforce. ADC, another New Deal program, had its roots in late nineteenth-century understandings of white family and gender roles that imagined welfare as replacing the income normatively earned by a white male breadwinning husband. ADC benefits were denied to poor households in which an adult male was present. Until the Civil and Welfare Rights movements of the 1960s, ADC benefits were also denied to black mothers, since it was expected that they would work regardless of marital status.[18] By the mid-1990s, many middle-class white women had entered the workforce, leading to criticism of a program that allowed poor women to receive benefits without working.[19]

In 1996, Congress and President Clinton ended AFDC through the Personal Responsibility and Work Opportunity Reconciliation Act (PRWORA), a law more commonly known as "welfare reform." PRWORA replaced AFDC with a program called Temporary Aid to Needy Families (TANF), which provides temporary financial assistance while requiring recipients' participation in work programs.[20] It also funds job training and child care to support welfare-leavers, though funding for these programs has never been enough to meet increased needs. TANF job training programs typically focus on preparing women for low-wage jobs, rather than supporting the higher education or advanced skill training necessary for middle-class jobs. In the 20 years since welfare reform, poverty rates have not gone down. Instead of improving the lives of poor families, TANF created a large pool of low-wage workers. Many home care workers are drawn from welfare-to-work programs that offer employers tax incentives to place TANF recipients in jobs.

While US poverty, health care, and aging policies created a racialized direct care workforce, international economic policies create transnational webs of care. Since the 1990s, neoliberal economic policies around the world have created widespread economic dislocation. This led to extensive international migration as workers from poorer countries seek new ways to earn money to support families at home. Women form a significant portion of these migrants. Female migrants are often limited to domestic and care jobs in part because their educational credentials and work experience are not recognized in receiving countries like the United States. Sociologist Mary Romero notes that in the United States, domestic work has long been thought of as suitable labor for immigrant women and women of color because "workers were thought to benefit from the opportunity to be 'modernized'" through their exposure to the daily lives of wealthier white households.[21] As a consequence, immigrant women, like US-born women of color, fill a disproportionate share of domestic and direct care jobs.

Contemporary racial and gendered divisions of caring labor in the United States are a discriminatory inheritance stretching back to the founding of the nation, as shown by this brief history. From state-sanctioned slavery through welfare reform and the companionship exemption, federal law and public policy generate social conditions in which providing care for pay remains an important means of survival for women of color. This history is the unspoken framework of home care workers' life histories, shaping the choices available to them. Out of this restrictive structure, home care workers and their families creatively craft strategies of survival, infusing struggle with pride.

Home care workers' labor is (at least) doubly generative—making possible both the lives of older clients and their own kin. Home care workers not only learn how to care among kin, their obligations to kin motivate them to provide paid care. Despite the diversity of their backgrounds and experiences, the home care workers I met all spoke of becoming a home care worker as first and foremost a way to care for their own kin and households in the face of economic insecurity. In this way, their lives echo the arguments of black feminist sociologist Patricia Hill Collins, who wrote that while physical survival is often assumed for white middle-class children, struggles to foster the survival of families and communities of color "comprise a fundamental dimension of racial ethnic women's motherwork." In working for the survival of their families and communities, mothers of color regularly do more than their fair share of this generative labor, submerging individual autonomy and growth for the benefit of the group.[22] Like their mothers and grandmothers before them, many parlayed caregiving skills learned at home into an economic life raft, sustaining multiple generations of kin through their long hours of care work outside their homes. Their expertise as carers formed the foundation of both survival and moral imagination—it became one ground upon which they evaluated their own and others' moral value and social worth.

Keep Your Trade

As far back as she could remember, Doris had big plans and even bigger dreams. Though few of those dreams had come to pass by the time we met, Doris continued to use all the resources she could muster to move a little closer to her goals. She was born in the mid-1950s to working-class black parents in a rural county seat about a hundred miles from Memphis, Tennessee. Doris's family followed her father, a construction worker, from their hometown to Memphis and then to Jackson, where Doris graduated from high school. After Doris graduated from high school, her parents bought a house in their hometown, where her mother continued to live after her father's death.

As a young child, Sunday had been the highlight of Doris's week. After attending church in the morning with her parents, siblings, and paternal grandparents, they feasted—sometimes as a family and more often with the whole church community. Her grandmother, a school teacher, would cook greens and cornbread and ham and chicken dressing and potato salad and slaw and dinner rolls, all from scratch. Doris spoke wistfully of those church picnics, remembering that there would be "so much food there, it would be like a grocery store full of food. We ain't talkin' about two hams, we're talking about six, seven, eight hams. They would barbecue a whole pig. We're talking major food." Through these weekly feasts, kin and community nourished one another with spiritual and material care.

Growing and preparing food infused Doris's memories of that time. Doris learned to play her role generating the life of the family by learning to care for livestock and prepare the inexpensive, labor-intensive dishes that filled the family's larder. Her parents had a farm where she remembered taking care of the animals when she was "real, real young . . . We used to milk cows. I used to do the chickens. We had 200 chickens on that yard. I used to go in the big hen house and get the eggs. Like my chore. I didn't like it, but once I got used to it and thought about it, it was fun." Her memories were deeply sensory, shaping her tastes and preferences in the present. Doris spoke at length of long summer afternoons spent with her grandmother, learning to preserve all kinds of food, things like black-eyed peas, butter beans, green beans, and homemade jam. Doris's grandmother also taught her how to slaughter, clean, and butcher a hog, and how to make chitlins and head cheese from the meat.[23] Doris wistfully recalled learning to make homemade sour buttermilk, which was much more delicious than anything she could purchase in Chicago-area stores.

These lessons were Doris's inheritance, meant to pass along family culinary traditions, and critical economic skills. Multiple generations of her family emphasized the survival value of building a diverse set of skills. She recalled, "My father said that, my grandfather said that, my grandmother said that, 'always keep your way to make you some money in order to survive.' They told me the name of the game to survive. Don't always try to have one thing and you can't do nothing else." These lessons remained invaluable, she said, because "if push comes to shove, if I lose my job today, I can get in a kitchen and make some homemade jam . . . take peaches, pears, or anything I can get to buy a bushel. Start me with enough money to buy a bushel, can that stuff, sell it . . . it's always like, keep your trade. That was the name of my family . . . that's the way I was raised. We weren't rich. . . . I've never been hungry, never been with no place to stay. I had family, but my parents was strict and they were down on [formal] education. They'd say, you got to know this, because society. If you miss this, society will eat you up." Her choice of metaphor was uncanny, nearly literal—to avoid being cannibalized by society, she would have to sustain herself and others with the foods of her childhood. To avoid getting eaten up by society, Doris's kin taught her to transform their generative labor into a trade.

During these family lessons in domestic food production and the pragmatics of survival, Doris began to dream of a professional career quite different from the practical working-class trades her parents and grandparents favored. Her comfort with the grisly, bloody, and physically demanding process of turning living animals into food inspired her desire to become a doctor. She remembered, "I always wanted to be a doctor, especially after doing all that chitlin'ing, because I had seen everything! Blood don't bother me . . . I've been in all kinds of slaughterhouses. I get it. I worked it. I learned how to purify the meat." From the bloody, smelly work of butchering it did not seem like such a stretch for Doris to imagine facing the similarly bloody but more prestigious and lucrative work of doctoring instead.

Until her family moved to Jackson, Doris attended segregated schools. Her grades were never very good, even though she had always been a "book person . . . always interested in why this works, why this works, and how come this is like this." Her father was wary of Doris's bookishness and medical ambition, counseling her about the importance of street smarts. He occasionally grounded her for "staring at a book too long." In ninth grade, a teacher at her integrated high school noticed that Doris's written work did not match her knowledge and had her tested for dyslexia. With appropriate accommodations, Doris's grades rose quickly.

After high school, Doris planned to enter the air force, hoping to gain medical training through her military service. A spleen injury and three-month hospital stay thwarted that plan. Instead, Doris got a job working with her mom at a textile factory and started saving money for college. After visiting her aunt in Wisconsin on vacation, Doris decided to move north. She took a job at the factory where her aunt worked, hoping to save enough money to register for pre-med classes at a nearby university. She had two daughters, a few years apart, which made her even more determined to pursue her education and make a better life for all of them.

Doris continued taking classes while her children were young, relying on a combination of scholarships and AFDC to make ends meet. It was 1990, and under the welfare rules of the time, it hadn't been easy to convince the welfare officers to pay for child care while she went to school. She recalled, "They gave me a hard time and told me to wait until my kids got old enough to go to school. At first they weren't going to pay for my daycare and stuff. I had to fight them for that. If I had waited until my kids got old enough to go to school, I would have been behind trying to get my training that I got now. I fought both ways in getting the education." The welfare officers also tried to influence her private life, pushing her to marry the man that she dated and sometimes lived with. Welfare officers (and the politicians that wrote the laws those officers enforced) claimed that poor women would be better off building families according to white bourgeois kinship norms. Her boyfriend's job prospects were much worse than hers, and the idea that their marriage would raise her income enough to replace welfare benefits was laughable. As broad discourses of race and kinship continued to impinge on Doris's life, she pushed back. She insisted that investments in her education and career were her family's best path forward.

One of Doris's university science teachers suggested that she pursue training as a Certified Nursing Assistant (CNA). Doris recalled the instructor's advice as intended to offer her a more financially stable path through college to medical school: "He says, 'I'll tell you what you need to do. You got a long way to go.' He was talking about finance. I had two girls I was raising by myself and trying to go to school, he showed me the way to do that. He said, 'Take a break from this university and go to Tech college and do a CNA.' At that time CNA was only eight weeks. I could do that and work at the same time. That's what I did. He showed me the way to always continue, and that I had a long way to pay for, and how to do that when I have two kids. I'm glad I did that."[24] While pursuing a CNA was a quick path to lowering Doris's reliance on government benefits, in the long run it did not offer her nearly the same earning potential as would an undergraduate degree or other medical training.

Doris's training complemented what she learned from kin, improving the care she provided to both clients and family members. Doris saw the domestic skills and moral sentiments she had learned among her family as central to her caring work. At the same time, she valued the medical knowledge and professional health care skills she had gained from her CNA training. Having grown up close to her grandmother, Doris always enjoyed spending time with older adults and listening to their stories, so she quickly took to her new job as a nursing assistant. She also told stories of accurately diagnosing both family members and clients with severe illnesses before they had seen a doctor. Doris diagnosed her aunt at the onset of a serious stroke by sight alone, haranguing reticent relatives to call an ambulance. She proudly recalled that, "The doctor told her [aunt] that if it wasn't for me, she was walking dead. My medical field that I've been so stubborn about from childhood has been paying off. I never did make it to being a doctor, but I'm so close." She used expertise in cooking and keeping house to sustain the homes of her clients, and she used her formal health care training to diagnose and save the lives of her kin.

Doris felt ongoing tension between providing financially for her daughters and being available to parent them in other ways. For 16 years, she lived with a man she sometimes called her "common law husband." He never supported her or her daughters financially. It proved impossible to spend so much of her time and energy sustaining the lives of others through her care work and still create for her children the life she wanted. After finishing CNA training she found a good job at a nursing home. It paid well and offered good health insurance, a rarity for CNA jobs. The job regularly demanded long hours—16-hour shifts and 80-hour weeks. For the first time, she could make ends meet financially, and was proud that she could support her daughters. The grueling hours were not without costs, however, both to her family and her health.

One afternoon, as I dusted Mr. Thomas's floorboards and she scrubbed his bathroom, Doris told me about the cost she found hardest to bear. "My daughter is very depressed and she makes me depressed. She needs counseling real bad but the system won't let me help her . . . she was raped." Given the awkward setting, Doris didn't say much more, except that she attributed her daughter's ongoing instability to her earlier rape. Later, when we sat down to record her life history, she told me more of what had happened when her daughter was "like thirteen, fourteen, somewhere around there. I was at work. I was at work all the time those days. So my stepson had been coming around all the time—he didn't live with us no more, but he was around." She was at work when she got "a call from my aunt who was watching the girls saying that I have to come home right away because there was a problem." She took a deep breath, "My aunt had found my daughter crying in the bathtub, girl wouldn't stop sobbing. Finally, we got her to tell us what happened—my stepson had told her to do things and had touched her privates. I dunno why she didn't just tell me—maybe she felt guilty, or embarrassed. I always told the girls they could talk about sex with me, taught them all the right names for their parts. . . . I just didn't know what to do."

Doris attributed her daughter's subsequent difficulties to this assault, saying, "She's always had problems, since then, all kinds. A year later, ran away. Stayed gone two weeks, came home pregnant." Doris sighed, "I always told the girls, condom, everything about sex. I bought boxes, cases of condoms. I told them not to get pregnant, that I'd put them out on the curb." Doris continued, "So she was scared to death that I'd do that, but I wouldn't. So she called, talked to her sister to see if she could come back home. She came home and lived with me and went back to school. Baby went to daycare; I made public aid pay for that too. I was working two jobs." Her daughter struggled ever since. She ran with a "bad crowd," and struggled with addiction. She spent time in prison. Doris tried to get her daughter into treatment, but the system offered fewer beds for rehabilitation than prison.

Though Doris was not one for regrets, she still felt guilty that her long work hours had left her unable to protect her daughter. In this telling of her history, Doris laid bare the limits of her capacity to generate the lives of others. Doris' defensiveness belied both her guilt and her anger. She had given her daughters the sexual education she believed would protect them. She worked two jobs to keep a roof over their heads. What more should she have done? Ultimately, that she had to work so many hours just to pay the bills was confirmation that, as her kin had told her, "society will eat you up."

With the birth of her grandchild, Doris worked to sustain the life of yet another generation. But she could only stretch so far. The long hours also took a serious toll on Doris's health, eventually compromising her ability to work much at all. About 12 years before we met, "stuff got messed up and went haywire." After years working long hours, her joints started hurting. At first, Doris thought she had a cold and blamed it on exhaustion. But then, as she recalled, "the pain I had in my bones, it was just like my soul, like my skeleton was infected, burning like it was a fire that wouldn't go out." She coped for months by taking about eight pills of Advil a day. Then, one snowy day in February, a circular bruise emerged on her skin, which looked "just like a sidewalk burn, and it was raw . . . at first I put a patch on it and went to work and I was sick. That day, I was sick." Doris was still at work when she began "constantly throwing up." She was sweaty and hyperventilating. Her blood pressure fell rapidly. She initially tried to recuperate alone in a bathroom at the nursing home. She grew so weak she had to pull the emergency cord meant for the residents. She was barely able to unlock the door for the nurse who came to help her. Recalling that day, she described a harrowing scene in which the nurses kept her from fainting by opening the window so the frigid air could revive her.

At the hospital, she was given anti-inflammatory medication to help with her joint pain, but nothing improved. Her boss at the nursing home told her not to return to work until she found out what was really wrong with her. They put her on disability leave so that she could receive insurance payments. After many months of doctors' appointments, she was finally diagnosed with lupus. An autoimmune disease, lupus is often precipitated by exhaustion and stress. The doctor prescribed very strong steroids and told her to take an entire year off of work. She recalled that the doctor "wouldn't even let me exercise for over a year, and then he told me I had workaholic disease." Doris had spent thousands of hours generating the life of others. Yet for Doris, paid care work also generated illness that had crept into her weary bones and aching muscles.

Woven through Doris's narrative were multiple, competing understandings of kinship, care, and obligation shaping Doris's life and hopes for the future. From kin she learned the sensorial skills and moral commitments to sustaining life and kinship, turning them into a trade. Kin also taught her to work hard to ensure her survival and that of her children. Doris worked herself sick to live up to these familial and national ideologies of kinship, obligation, and care.

Unable to work, to "keep her trade," Doris was again forced to rely on public assistance. Again, she turned to the survival skills she had learned while raising her children. She drew all of her disability insurance from the nursing home before she began receiving disability insurance from the federal Social Security Insurance (SSI) program. After a year, she went back to work in the nursing home. She soon realized that working there was too physically strenuous, as she continued to have recurrent episodes of severe pain due to her lupus. Finally, she left the nursing home altogether and began doing home care. She worked as many hours as she could manage, but it was far less than she had worked at the nursing home.

Several years later, when I met Doris, she had lost her house in Wisconsin and relocated to a Chicago suburb located about an hour from the city. I never learned exactly what happened to provoke these changes. Doris hinted that her partner had cheated on her and had not been paying his share of the bills, causing her to lose the house. He continued to call her. She refused to take him back. No longer able to work grueling 16-hour days due to her lupus, she still received SSI benefits. She could not make ends meet on her SSI income alone, so she worked part time for Belltower, where she earned just above the minimum wage.[25]

During the time I knew her, Doris lived in a small one-bedroom apartment. She kept the windows closed, the curtains drawn tight, and the air conditioning turned as high as she could afford during the summer. The sunlight and heat set off lupus flares. She shared the apartment with Janice and Teshawn (her younger daughter and grandson). Together the two women were just barely able to make ends meet.

Doris was passing on her trade, just as her forbears had passed on theirs. Doris was proud that Janice had recently started working as a CNA. She was pleased that Janice "passed her test before she went to class because I told her everything that was going to happen." She taught both Janice and me that care required both moral imagination and embodied skill. She recalled, "I told her [Janice] the same thing I told you. 'If you don't care about these people, don't do it.' You'll do more for a person that needs your help because when you get that same age and you need some help, you hope you can get the same respect. . . . Just like you have a newborn baby and you're going to cherish that baby. You don't want nothing to happen so that's the way you're going to treat an elderly person. You're going to give them the same respect." Janice had worried she would be disgusted by bodily care, and asked how to handle the sensory aspects of the job. Doris recalled the conversation beginning with Janice asking: "'What if they shit all over themselves?' Well, I said, 'You clean them up.' She said, 'I can't stand the smell.' I said, 'You get used to it. You smell yourself, don't you? You can do it." At the time we spoke, Janice was still working at a nearby nursing home, prompting Doris to say that her lessons "worked, didn't it!".

While passing down the expertise she inherited from her own mother and grandmother, Doris also passed down the forms of moral imagination developed over years as a paid care worker. In recounting—and passing on—these lessons to her daughter and me, Doris moved seamlessly between practical and moral instruction, for they were one and the same. For Doris, the bodily discipline required to manage disgust was one more form of the broader moral imagination required to care well for others. Whether it was a matter of respect or cleaning shit, Doris argued that a good care worker should treat an older person as a future version of themselves, or their own child.[26] Though racism, poverty, and limited options had funneled her into home care, she nevertheless saw this work as a choice that imposed deep moral obligations. Those who did not care about vulnerable people should not work in these jobs. From her childhood experiences learning to cook among kin to teaching her daughter the moral imagination needed to navigate the sensorial challenges of care work, Doris was passing on her inheritance.

Without both generations' caring labor within and outside their home, Doris's whole precarious household would fall apart. Her decade-old Oldsmobile could break down, her lupus could flare, her eldest daughter could be arrested. With no economic savings, any setback was likely to cause a cascade of problems, costing them their apartment or her job. Doris worried that if she were no longer able to work in home care, she would be unable to care for her family. Her care work sustained the lives of her clients, but for her family these overlapping and interdependent forms of care generated a precarious kind of life.

Doris's family had intentionally passed on to her a variety of survival skills and moral values that became the foundation of her approach to care work. Though Grace Washington also developed her approach to care among kin, her skills were not the result of an intentional inheritance. Instead, Grace's approach to homemaking grew out of her attempts to protect her kin and create stability amid a home torn by violence.

A Home-knitted Person

Ever since she was a teenager, Grace saw care and protection as deeply intertwined. She carried this ethic into her paid care work. Grace was expert at generating life amid hardship and violence, and at turning her home into a sanctuary. She extended her ability to create sanctuaries to her elderly clients. As Grace spoke about her own history and her ethic of care, she returned again and again to the vulnerability and sanctity of homes—whether her paying clients' or her own. For Grace, caring for homes was essential to caring for persons.

The youngest of six children, Grace had been caring for people since she was a teenager. Her parents both worked long hours to keep a roof over their heads. After coming north from Mississippi, her parents settled in Chicago, where her mother found work at one of the automobile factories and her father was a carpenter. As she remembered it, "my background was kind of hard, because my dad at first was an abusive father. He would fight my mother all the time. I would wonder how did she get the strength, how could she constantly do it and had six kids and them come in not knowing if she was going to have a fight or not." Grace recalled that she drew "strength from my mother. My other sisters, they would be doing their own thing, so I would just be around the house to help and make things better for my mother until it just became a ritual for me." From an early age, she "was sitting there on the washing machine or sitting on the kitchen sink watching my mama cook and watching my mama how she takes care of the house. That's just something I wanted to do. I'm like 'Mama, one day when I get grown, I'm going to be a nurse.' I ain't quite got there yet." Grace understood nursing as a professional form of the skills she had learned at her mother's side. She saw her home care work and pursuit of nursing as the continuation of a path begun at her mother's apron strings.

As a young girl, Grace hoped that by caring for her parents' home she might protect her mother from her father's wrath. She recalled, "If the house wasn't kept up, I didn't want my daddy to jump on my mama and say, 'Dinner ain't cooked and the house ain't clean.'" As soon as she was old enough she started to do "stuff around the house and clean up. By the time she come in, I had the house cleaned from front to back. Everybody's clothes was washed and dinner was on the table at five o'clock every day." By the time she was 15, Grace was taking full care of the house. She described herself from the time she was young as "an old-fashioned kind of gal. . . . I'm a home-knitted person. I've been like that all my life." Her commitment to home linked her youth and her work, seeing both as methods of generating and protecting the lives of others. Grace understood her commitment to sustaining the lives of others as a form of spiritual worship. She told me that besides spending time at home, "the only thing I really like to do is go to church and I love to sing and I love playing gospel music. I admire the way my mother would work and take care of the house." For Grace, homes, like churches, were places that nurtured what she considered traditional and non-materialistic values.

Grace and her husband shared a deep love of home and desire to care for those around them. Grace compared herself to her sisters, who were outgoing as youths, and became single mothers at young ages. She intentionally waited until her mid-twenties, after she met her husband, to start a family. She described their shared love of home and desire to care for those around them as given "by the grace of God. He instilled in my heart and in my soul a daily ritual with me. I could see a stranger in the street and if that person is mean or something, I can help them, or if someone is hurt. Fortunately, my husband was raised pretty much with the same environment." Grace was profoundly protective of her household, only expanding it when she met a partner as committed as she was to a spiritual and domestic life.

Marriage expanded Grace's experiences of care. Her husband had his own health problems, and she saw it as her responsibility to "keep him up and his heart tickering good and his blood sugar down." Helping him manage his diabetes had proven useful in her work. She learned how to adjust recipes and substitute ingredients to manage diabetic patients. She could also count on her husband to care for her, "when I'm tired or when I need to be taken care of, he finds the strength to care for me. . . . I thought it was just fairy tales that you will meet somebody that is totally right and compatible. Like bull crap. Just too good to be true. But it's true." She continued, "If you are ever fortunate enough to find your soul mate, you do what you got to do to keep it going and keep doing that so the soul mate is happy. You don't let no one or nothing come into your household." The protective ethic Grace developed in her parents' household extended to the home she created with her husband, and she was wary of intrusion by anyone who might harm their happiness. Grace harbored a gentle disdain for her clients' kin, who invited virtual strangers into their households, seemingly without concern about the danger this might pose to their loved ones. Her commitment to caring for clients was driven partly by her concerns that they were not adequately cared for or protected by their kin.

Grace transformed everyday care and domestic skill into a kind of familial shield. As a parent, Grace protected her own household and children in much the same way she had protected her mother. After Grace and her husband had children, she started looking for a way to help support their family economically. Her husband was an experienced auto mechanic and worked odd jobs, but chronic illness prevented him from working full time. Seeking a source of income, she turned the domestic skills her mother had taught her into a full-time occupation that enabled her to actively care for her children. Grace framed the story of how she came to paid home care work as a kind of personal origin story, the story of how she came to be. She recalled, "I started out doing home care because when I had my children I refused to take them to a babysitter because during that time they was fondling kids and you couldn't trust nobody at that time. So I'm like no, I had these babies and I'm going to stay here and take care of these babies."[27] She decided that, "When I go to work, I'm going to get me a job where I can work around my kids. So an older lady upstairs where I used to live told me that I could get a job doing home care service. I'm like 'what is home care service?' You just go to the senior's house and take care of them." Grace remembered thinking, "Yeah. That's something that I can get into. That is something I can sort of relate to. She got me into it and I've been doing it ever since. This has been since my babies were young, and now my son is in college. . . . That's where I'm at and that's how I came to be." Generating and protecting the life of her kin by generating and protecting the lives of elderly clients had made Grace what and where she was in life.

Working in home care meant becoming a transient part of her clients' households. Grace initially took home care jobs as a way of keeping her own household safe. It was the only job she knew of where she could earn a living, protect her family, and honor the gifts she felt had been given to her by God. Grace spoke of learning the skills to care well from her mother, but credited God with giving her the temperament and endurance to care well. "I can't do what I do on my own. It's something within. The Lord gives me the strength to do what I do and I don't know what it is about me, it's just some kind of way I have of dealing with people. I never met a person yet that I have not dealt with. . . . I praise the Man and I hope he keeps it going for me. Once I get into the mode and get into what I do, I do it as if I'm doing it in my own house." Grace extended her commitments to her own household to those of her clients, such that her understandings of kinship became the basis of her paid care.

Grace kept her clients' homes with the same pride she kept her own, trying to make them places in which elders would feel safe, happy, and comfortable. She told me that when supervisors told her a new client was "one of the grouchy ladies, I'm like well, that's what you say. Let me go in there. Give me two days with her and I bet you when I leave there, they going to be like 'Wow. What did you do?' I didn't do nothing. I just go look and observe and in some kind of way the Father puts a certain light on me whereas I see certain things." Grace drew on her faith and her lifetime caring for kin. She saw her role as becoming whomever her clients needed. She said, "I'm so persistent that I'm not going to let you sit there and wallow in your misery because misery loves company and I ain't trying to be your company. I'm going to be your friend, sister, brother. If you need a hug, I'll give you hug. I'll be whatever you need me to be." Grace saw her empathic skill to become whatever kind of person her clients needed her to be as a spiritual gift that connected her domestic life with her clients' lives. By treating clients as members of her extended household, Grace was able to put herself in the role of whichever kind of kin they seemed to need. In considering their homes her home, she extended the model of domestic protection and comfort she had learned caring for her own kin to her paying clients.

When I met Grace, both of her children were grown and out of the house. She was working longer hours than ever before. She remained the primary caregiver to at least two other generations of kin: her parents and her grandchildren. Her son was studying pre-medicine on a scholarship at a college in Florida. Midway through the time I knew Grace, her daughter was arrested. Grace swooped in to care for her granddaughter, terrified that Child Protective Services (CPS) would otherwise take custody of the child.

For nearly a decade, Grace had also been taking care of her father, now blind and suffering from diabetes. She stopped to see him nearly every day on her way home from work. Other family members had little contact with him because of his abusive history, but she had come to view him as vulnerable and in need of protection. She said, "I got to taking care of my dad, you know . . . my sisters and them won't even go around him because they still resent him for what he did to my ma and I'm still like well, he's still our dad. He's blind. The Lord is punishing him for his sins and what he's done so I'm not going to sit over here and let him suffer because of what he did in the past." Grace continued, "Right now my dad is my best friend. . . . I go there to do the cooking, the laundry, and get everything that he needs in there." After his glaucoma diagnosis a decade earlier, she rearranged his apartment to keep him safe. She said, "I have it set up whereas he's blind, and that man walk around there like he got eyes. Yes, he do. Everything is in just the right place . . . I go in there and cook his dinner fresh because he don't like too much street food and he don't like them frozen dinners. I got the Tupperware things and I pre-package him meals. . . . I've been doing it ever since faithfully. I don't know where I get the strength."

Grace told me that she cared for her clients much as she cared for her father—accepting their histories and their challenging personalities. She focused on becoming whom the other person needed her to be, not on what she needed from them. In caring for her father, this meant coming to peace with his abusive history and his alcoholism. She explained, "We'll talk about the past and stuff and why he do what he did or whatever. He was drinking alcohol and alcohol plays a lot into it. He's been drinking all his life. He don't drink every day, but he's like 'If you stop me from drinking, you're going to kill me.' This is what he truly believes. Like I said, I'm not trying to change you, I'm not trying to give you my rules or regulations. I'm going to do what makes you happy and what you feel comfortable with. Simple as that." Toward the end of this statement, Grace referred indirectly to her conflicts with Belltower supervisors over how to care for one of their clients. The supervisor wanted Grace to force the client onto a strict daily routine. Grace resisted, insisting that doing so would confuse and upset her client.[28] Making sure her clients were happy and comfortable was more important to Grace than official rules. Drawing on the models of kinship and care learned throughout her life, Grace saw her role as protecting clients' households and relationships from outside threats so that they would live comfortably in old age.

Grace hoped that her care, good care, would generate a peaceful, happy, comfortable life for her clients, her kin, and herself. The desire to protect her kin led her to paid home care in the first place. She always seemed just on the verge of achieving such a life—saving money to qualify for a subsidized program to purchase a house in a less dangerous neighborhood, taking online classes at night to train for a better job. Each time she would get close to one of these goals, something would happen. A car repair would deplete the savings, or family demands would make it impossible for her to finish her course.

Grace seemed to be constantly taking care of others—her clients, her father, her granddaughter, her husband. Though Grace could rely on the care and support of her husband, her paid work was their only steady source of income. Grace believed her care work should support the kind of stable, safe life she helped create for her clients. Instead, home care work enabled only a precarious form of life, one in which Grace and her kin always remained one crisis away from losing their car, losing their home, or losing their health.

Generating Care and Inequality

Amid systemic inequality, home care workers creatively manage the challenges of sustaining their families across generations, drawing on familial inheritances of domestic skills and moral imagination to make life possible for their own families and their elderly clients. Viewed in a vacuum, Doris's and Grace's stories might be seen as confirming some of the harshest stereotypes circulating in the United States about poor women and women of color. Unable to support their families despite working long hours, both relied on public benefits to make ends meet. Under current labor and welfare policies, women working in essential but underfunded fields like home care have little chance of ever earning enough to support their kin, thanks to the long legacies of discrimination inscribed into social and economic policy. These policies create and perpetuate fragmented, underfunded systems of elder care that depend on poor women of color who have little option but to work for low wages. Despite these low wages, both Doris and Grace spoke of themselves as morally committed to care that generated meaningful lives for their elderly clients.

Kin taught care workers these skills as part of passing on the arts of survival. Home care workers learned alongside kin the forms of generative labor required to sustain their families amid ongoing violence and hardship. In the process, workers were inculcated with a rich, sensory-laden, moral understanding of why and how they should care for themselves, for family, and for others in the community. These practices regenerated gendered divisions of labor within the family, qualifying daughters for evolving jobs in domestic service, while sons learned manual trades like carpentry and bricklaying. In these ways, the households in which workers had grown up shaped their senses of what women, homes, and care should be. When they entered paid care work, tensions arose between the moralities of care learned among kin and the demands of care in the marketplace.

For many workers, caring well for others was also an important moral and cultural value. Doris and Grace emphasized their expertise in elder care, perhaps to distinguish their work from other forms of domestic labor associated with subservience. Black domestic workers have a historically ambivalent relationship with paid care work. Patricia Hill Collins notes that, historically, black women have hoped their children would not follow them into domestic work. Collins shows that domestic workers typically taught their children "the value of their work as part of the ethics of caring and personal accountability" while also pushing children to seek more widely respected careers.[29] In focusing on their formal training as well as their inherited and God-given skill, Doris and Grace emphasized the essential role they played in generating meaningful lives for their elderly clients. Working for older, vulnerable adults enabled them to frame their work as a form of compassionate service rather than as coerced subservience.

Home care workers described themselves as moral and practical authorities by virtue of their commitments to care. In doing so, they continued a long tradition of domestic workers promoting the moral value of generative labor as a way of critiquing the low social and economic value attributed to this work.[30] Popular discourse in the United States often depicts care as a natural extension of women's biological capacities for reproduction. Implicitly racist discourses paint women of color and immigrant women as naturally better caregivers. Such discourses imagine women of color as racially and culturally closer to nature and less corrupted by the alienating effects of modernity. Care workers, on the other hand, narrated their capacity to care as a form of expertise that built on gendered inheritances. Sociologist Bonnie Thornton Dill argues that these kinds of moral arguments are themselves pragmatic survival strategies in a racist and sexist world. Without the workplace structures and protections available to other workers, domestic employers and employees focus on "personal traits: the employee's manner of speech or dress, her attitude and appearance, the employer's kindness and generosity" to evaluate one another. Though workers never lose awareness that they are entitled to a fair wage, Dill argues that they "also understood the nature of the occupation" and develop their "human relations skills, because [they] learned quickly that they would become important tools for survival."[31] For home care workers, moral imagination joins the other "human relations skills" Dill describes. To earn the trust of their employers and others, care workers present themselves not only as empathic, skilled, and reliable but also as morally—rather than only economically—committed to care.[32]

Home care workers recognized their skill at generative labor. They sought formal training that would enable them to work in health care professions commensurate with their abilities. Thanks to long legacies of racial and educational segregation, home care workers typically grew up in neighborhoods without quality schools. Limited resources and family responsibilities made it hard for them to complete lengthy and expensive training. Home care jobs require minimal formal training, implicitly relying on workers' kin to impart the moral understandings and embodied skills that enable them to provide empathic care to older adults. In this respect, home care agencies rely on the generative labor of workers' kin to lower costs and increase profitability in an intimate instantiation of capitalism's broader dependence on kinship relations.[33] Without support for further training, care workers are often unable to realize their aspirations of leveraging their expertise in care for more stable, better-paying jobs. In this way, the home care industry commodifies multiple forms of familial care while regenerating the precarious conditions that constantly threaten their families' survival.

Though policy makers and analysts draw sharp distinctions between unpaid family care and paid care, in the lives of home care workers, care-for-money and care-for-kin were inextricably intertwined, each making the other possible. Public policies assume that families will be able to economically and socially support the lives of young children, while offering inadequate support to families whose work does not alleviate their poverty. Care workers took jobs in home care to provide the financial support their families desperately need, relying on other (often older and/or disabled) kin to care for young children. Care workers appreciated the comparatively flexible schedules home care jobs allowed, but were often frustrated that they received no paid leave to care for kin, were rarely assigned regular hours, and had limited opportunities for career advancement. In this sense, care workers' personhood is only publicly recognized in limited ways, through their relations to their clients but not through their relations to kin.

Home care agencies harness the models of kinship and care that home care workers learn from their families, turning workers' inheritance into revenue. The transformation from care-for-kin to care-for-profit is tense and full of friction, and contributes to the ongoing constitution of social personhood for those involved. Though home care workers extend moral models of care from their own households to the households of their clients, a variety of agency and government policies and laws impose boundaries between these households. In the process, agencies constitute care workers and older Chicagoans as independent persons. Thus, even as workers' and clients' households are morally connected, agency rules compel supervisors to impose restrictions on the flow of money, goods, and sentiment between households. What should and should not travel between workers' lives and older adults' lives is a persistent question facing everyone involved in home care, to which I now turn.

3

Making Care Work

Training and Supervision in Home Care Agencies

The line for the restroom snaked out the door and down the hallway. More than 50 of us, all women but two, had been sitting in Plusmore Home Care's training room for nearly three hours. It was the first day of a weeklong training for new home care workers. We had been slowly draining jumbo coffee cups and soda bottles brought from home as Alicia Morgan, Plusmore's head trainer, made her way through the tedious business of getting us organized. In the bathroom line, women talked and chatted, making friends and comparing notes. "How'd you find out about this job?" "Have you been in home care before?" "Where do you live?" "Got kids?" I stood out, the only pale face in line. The woman in front of me asked me a few questions about my research project, trying to make sense of the vague description Alicia gave at the beginning of class. Other trainees ignored me.

Or at least they ignored me until I unknowingly broke an unspoken rule, committing one of those etiquette gaffes that anthropologists are famous for. After using the restroom, I washed my hands, walked to the paper towel dispenser, pulled a piece of towel, and dried my hands. I then threw the towel in the wastebasket and headed for the door across the long bathroom. As I walked across the room, I caught sight of the rolling eyes and looks of annoyance from the women still waiting in line, a few subtly shaking their heads in disapproval.

As I waited in line during the next break, I paid more attention to what other women were doing after they washed their hands. After drying their hands, each woman pulled an additional piece of paper towel. She then returned to the sink she had used and thoroughly wiped and dried it. They made sure there were no puddles remaining on the sink edge to soil the next user's blouse, no wayward splatters of soap that would dry onto the sink. Only then did they throw out their towels and leave the restroom.

How had all these other women known to wipe down their sinks and why had I not known to do the same? I was too embarrassed to ask other trainees, whom I did not know very well. I later asked the home care workers I came to know better if they followed this practice, and how they had learned it. None of them could pinpoint a specific lesson in this etiquette—they had never thought to do otherwise. They thought it was probably something they learned as children, watching their mothers and other women in their communities. Workers were surprised that I had not been similarly socialized. They spoke of wiping down the sink as a matter of basic courtesy. A few longtime workers told me that making a living cleaning up after other people made them conscientious about not leaving unnecessary messes behind for custodial staff. In bringing this ethic to the workplace, trainees also created a more pleasant environment for potential co-workers and saved their potential employer the money it might cost to clean a messier bathroom.

Home care agencies build upon women's familial experience of care while seeking to transform them into workers whose labor conforms to the ethical and temporal norms of American workplaces. Conflicts regularly arise between people's moral ideologies about care, the economic pressures of capitalist markets, and the laws that govern labor and elder care in the United States. By turning care into work, agencies justify their existence in the market as managing the predictable tensions that regularly arise in home care. Through their management practices, agencies struggle to reconcile contradictory understandings of caring labor. Agency staff navigate these tensions on a case-by-case basis. Supervisors' decisions have the improvisational quality of ongoing moral "tinkering" in that, as Annemarie Mol describes, they take it as inevitable that "different 'goods' reflecting not only different values but different ways of ordering reality" must be dealt with together.[1] This chapter traces the transformation of moral values into economic value by focusing on the everyday ethics practiced by home care agency management staff as they mediate between national moralities, the needs of their agencies, the needs of clients, and their own ethics.[2]

Home care agencies are one of many street-level organizations responsible for the day-to-day implementation of US welfare state policies. In the case of home care, private agencies are primarily responsible for implementing the elder care policies of Medicaid, state programs, and/or private insurance companies. As employers of low-wage workers, they also play a crucial role implementing welfare-to-work (also known as "workfare") policies. Political scientist Evelyn Brodkin argues that street-level organizations are crucial "mediators of both policy and politics."[3] Street-level workfare organizations often advance gendered models of citizenship that frequently fail to recognize women's generative labor among kin.[4]

Agency supervisors are an example of what sociologist Michael Lipsky called "street-level bureaucrats," meaning that they have significant discretion over how to interpret policies that have conflicting implications in complex situations.[5] In what follows, I examine how agency management staff and supervisors navigate the frictions between common ideologies of care, economic pressures, and legal regulations across a range of situations necessary to running a home care agency. These include hiring and training workers, recruiting clients, staffing cases, and managing conflicts between workers and clients. Supervisors are also responsible for enacting federal, state, and agency policies regarding employment and elder care. In exchange for this labor, frontline supervisors earned national median wages of $17.17 per hour, or annual median incomes of $35,710, in 2015.[6]

Home care agencies translate the fluid work of generating life into industrial standards of temporal efficiency.[7] Agencies require workers to enact their domestic expertise and moral imaginations of care within the bounds of proscribed care plans that can be remunerated by the hour. While care plans delineate clear tasks of specified duration, the actual pace required of care practices is deeply dependent on context. For example, cooking a meal can take five minutes or an hour depending on the dish, and the frequency with which an older person will need assistance with toileting cannot be easily predicted in advance. Yet agencies and their workers are paid by the hour and so necessary tasks must be accomplished within preordained time frames.

Within these temporal structures, agencies need workers to provide care that is deeply attuned to clients' lives but not problematically entangled in them. The demand that workers and older adults should maintain a professional, yet deeply intimate, relationship reveals the contradictions at the heart of post-industrial American ideologies of public and private. Such ideologies frame care as a paradigmatically private concern, ideally undertaken among those with long-standing affective, reciprocal, and kinship bonds, rather than for material gain. On the other hand, public-sphere relationships are understood as characterized by impersonal, rational market exchanges and the rule of law. Within public moral norms, labor should be clearly defined and compensated by a wage. In actual practice, of course, affective bonds regularly shape business relationships just as family life involves material calculation. Workers are expected to care for clients with the kind of commitment and attunement they would show kin, but are also expected to see themselves as separate from their clients' lives and social relations.

Supervisors' practices and agency policies instantiate older adults and home care workers as independent both from one another and from broader social relations. Home care agencies treat employees and clients as having distinct roles in paid care relationships: workers provide care while clients receive it. This requires that agencies and their management staff morally imagine both older adults and workers as separable from complex reciprocal webs of care in which they both give and receive. It is common that workers and older adults try to include one another in these broader webs, yet doing so often creates problematic entanglements and disagreements. Supervisors respond to these conflicts by trying to draw boundaries that limit long-standing and emergent reciprocities in home care.[8]

The kinds of problems that arose at Belltower and Plusmore were similar, however the two agencies faced a somewhat different set of pressures due to their different funding sources. Both agencies were committed to their elderly clients' independence. However, they emphasized different aspects of this value and thus treated their clients and workers as somewhat different kinds of persons.

Plusmore's business depended on satisfying the terms of its contract with the state of Illinois. As public services are increasingly privatized, a growing number of street-level bureaucrats work for government contractors like Plusmore rather than for the government itself. This adds a level of complexity to supervisors' jobs, as they seek to implement public policy while maximizing their employers' revenues (and often profits). Plusmore negotiated its $13 per hour reimbursement rate with the state of Illinois, and had to offer services at a rate competitive with other area providers, most of which were non-profit. The contract required the agency to provide 40 hours of pre-employment training and additional quarterly in-service training to all workers. Plusmore workers, like other CCP care workers, were unionized by the SEIU, which consistently pressured the state to raise wages. As a result, Plusmore's wages for CCP services ranged from $7.65 to 9.15 per hour, depending on seniority. From its state reimbursement, Plusmore also paid for training, management, and administrative staff, insurance, office space, and a number of other costs. To oversee its 2,500-CCP-client caseload and 1,500 care workers, Plusmore employed approximately 12 supervisors and a handful of additional administrative and supervisory staff. The agency's administrators told me that the company earned about a penny of profit per hour of care the agency provided. Plusmore management was under constant pressure to make sure that it provided every contracted hour of care and retained large caseloads in order to satisfy corporate earnings goals and stockholders.

Belltower depended on customer satisfaction and word of mouth to stay in business. In privately funded agencies like Belltower, supervisors try to simultaneously satisfy customers while also adhering to a variety of legal and ethical demands. Supervisors faced ongoing pressure to attract and maintain enough clients to pay for the agency's operations. The agency charged $18–20 per hour of care, and paid workers around $6.75 per hour. Agency administrators explained that besides paying for wages, client fees paid for supervisors' wages, insurance, office space, and a variety of administrative costs. Though the gap between client fees and worker wages was much larger at Belltower, the additional money was used primarily to provide more attentive supervision. Belltower employed approximately eight supervisors and directors to oversee the agency's 250-client caseload. With smaller individual caseloads, supervisors offered much more intensive engagement with clients and workers. Belltower supervisors got to know their clients, enabling them to tailor care to specific clients' needs. As a non-profit organization, any revenue Belltower generated beyond its direct expenses helped to fund the larger elder care organization with which Belltower was affiliated.

Agencies' different funding sources affect how they imagine and generate their clients' independence. At Plusmore, state procedures and laws emphasized the rational, equitable distribution of resources based on an objective, universally applied measurement of need. Publicly funded care policies view older adults as liberal persons whose needs can be objectively evaluated as distinct from their broader social relations. As a result, publicly funded care instantiates older adults as independent persons in a democratic state in which rights and services are the result of citizenship and need rather than social position. At Belltower, on the other hand, older adults' independence was authorized by their privileged position as consumers who were entitled to purchase the services they desired. As consumers with economic freedom, Belltower clients' subjective tastes and preferences determined the kinds and quantity of care they received. Their independence was not the result of fair treatment by an ostensibly equitable state, but rather by their ability to wield economic power.

The ways that publicly and privately funded agencies construct clients' independence generate multiple gradients of inequality and power for older adults and workers. Public agencies, governed by notions of independence that emphasize equality, aim to treat each client in the same way. In the public-agency model, workers and clients are equally subjects of a democratic state, though they play different roles within that state. Private agencies, governed by notions of independence that emphasize consumer privilege, aim to treat clients the way they want to be treated. In this model, workers are not equal subjects, but rather subservient producers of purchased services. In both the publicly and privately funded models of care, workers' generative labor is extracted from their domestic and familial networks for the benefit of agencies and clients. Their families are never considered as part of paid home care work. The privately funded ethic of consumer privilege aligns more closely with the ways older adults morally imagine care. The agencies' different interpretations of independence create perceived hierarchies in the quality of care; good care goes to those who can pay for it.

"You Can't Be in It for the Money"

Training started at 8 a.m. sharp on Monday morning. As the clock hit the hour, Alicia Morgan, Plusmore Home Care's head trainer, took attendance. She spoke loudly over the excited murmur of trainees introducing themselves to one another. Fifty new trainees and I sat at rows of long, narrow tables. Except for me, every person in the room appeared to be African American. Perhaps a dozen appeared to be in their late teens or twenties, but most were decidedly middle-aged. The two men in the room joked lightly about being outnumbered by women. Alicia gathered Social Security numbers and identification documents from each trainee. She would later use the documents she collected to run criminal background checks on each aspiring home care worker.

According to Alicia, taking attendance and gathering identification documents were the two most important activities of the day, and to some extent, of the entire training program. Of the 50 people who started training that morning, fewer than 40 would remain on Friday afternoon. Some would not return on Tuesday, having realized that their criminal records would prevent them from ever being hired by Plusmore. Each day our numbers would shrink a little more, as trainees struggled to find consistent transportation and child care. The attendance policy was strict—anyone who did not show up promptly at 8 in the morning for each of the five days of training would not be hired. There was no point in continuing to attend, but some might try again when the next training session started two weeks later. As Alicia explained, anyone who could not arrive on time to training for five days in a row could not be relied upon to show up consistently to care for vulnerable elders.

With attendance taken, Alicia proceeded to describe Plusmore's organizational chart, focusing on the layers of management that workers would have the most contact with—the service coordinators who supervised workers and the quality assurance staff who conducted semi-annual home visits to monitor workers. Indirectly but efficiently, in that first half-hour of training, Alicia communicated that trainees were entering into hierarchical labor relations and began exercising the corporation's disciplinary power over workers' bodies and bodily habits. These "housekeeping tasks"—attendance, background checks, organizational charts—may not have been official training lessons, but they were central practices in the process of transforming trainees into home care workers.

With the initial organizational work completed, Alicia announced that the first official lesson of the training program was watching a short video. She wheeled a cart holding a 30-inch television to the front of the room and dimmed the lights. Produced by the Illinois Department of Aging, it was presumably a common feature in the training programs of many of the agencies that the state contracted to provide publicly funded home care. I'd like to say we strained to watch the video. But at barely 8:30 on a Monday morning, most of us were more concerned with our coffee and cell phones than with catching every word of the less-than-gripping film.

The film was intended to illustrate home care workers' job descriptions. In the process, the film promoted a particular moral orientation to care work that reflected common American ideologies of care as selfless and motivated by the moral desire to produce another's independence rather than by a carer's own material needs. The film promoted older adults as having unique social value because of their histories of experience, and asserted that helping elders remain at home was itself a way of maintaining their independence. In the film's opening scene, a female narrator read five guidelines in a slow, careful voice as the words appeared on screen: (1) The client's needs come first; (2) The family is your support team; (3) Never take sides in arguments; (4) Work to gain trust; and (5) Refer problems to your supervisor. In the next scene, a woman appeared on screen dressed in scrubs. To be a good care worker, she announced, "you can't be in it for the money. You have to enjoy what you are doing." Another woman appeared on screen dressed in a jacket and blouse, describing the great pride and satisfaction home care workers feel for their work. In part, she narrated, this is because home care workers help older adults remain in their own homes and "we all want to be at home, stay home, no matter our age. Our home is our castle." She described how workers would receive a care plan to follow with their clients, but "we" cannot go into clients' homes and abruptly tell them how it is. Rather, she said, workers must listen to clients' stories, because they are living historians and their stories are interesting. Home care workers, she continued, are very special people because the work can be very difficult and not everyone has the patience to do it. Still, seeing a smile on a client's face can make all the work worth it. In a later scene, an older person identified as a home care client described the importance of home care workers, saying, "you get involved in each other's life. It is caring, it is rewarding to the worker. I believe that for everyone who has a worker, caring comes to form some kind of love."

This video was the first formal description of home care work trainees encountered. The video spent very little time describing *how* workers might go about their jobs, or the practical, social, and emotional skills they would need to work successfully in older adults' homes. Though 50 adults had showed up at a sterile office building Monday morning at 8 a.m. to be trained for a new job, the video told them that they should not be motivated by a desire for material gain. Instead, the film framed several of the key contradictions of home care work as naturalized social relationships. First, in uncritically reproducing the common metaphor of private homes as their inhabitants' "castles," the film promoted the notion that the primary value of home care was that it allowed older adults to maintain autonomous control over their surroundings and daily lives. At the same time, the film noted that workers and clients would become involved in each other's lives, forming deep affective bonds. In referring to "the family" as the worker's support team, the film focused only on the role of older adults' kin. The film thus oriented workers to build alliances with clients' kin while failing to mention the ongoing contributions and demands of workers' families. The film effectively communicated that home care work is in part comprised of unidirectional emotional and relational commitments. Workers were expected to become a part of their clients' lives and build strong bonds with them, though their clients were not expected to reciprocate these efforts. At the same time, workers were expected to follow the norms and rules of their clients' households.

At the end of the first day of training, Alicia had a worker read the Plusmore "Home Care Aide Code of Ethics" and then emphasized a few key rules (see figure 3.1). The code of ethics lists 15 things workers were not allowed to do, most of which draw clear boundaries separating older adults' and workers' material and social lives. After all the rules had been read out loud, Alicia clarified situations in which workers might be tempted to break the rules. For example, one rule prohibits workers from eating their clients' food or drink, except tap water. Alicia said that "even if a client offers you dinner, even if they insist, you can't eat it. You have to say 'no thank you.' If a client offers you a soda, say no. Many of our clients are on limited incomes. They want to be nice, they want to be good hosts, but they might not have enough to eat themselves." Alicia explained that the rule against sharing personal information with clients could be hard to follow, but was very important. She explained that it was the home care worker's job to "worry and care" for older adults. If clients knew too much about their workers, they might worry about them, or judge them. Either way it could complicate their relationships. Alicia further clarified that workers were not allowed to accept loans or gifts of any kind from clients, nor were they allowed to purchase anything from clients. "Sometimes clients or their family members will be selling something, like makeup from Avon or Mary Kay. You can't buy those. Don't buy anything from your clients, from their family. It can get messy and create problems for you." Alicia repeat-

HOME CARE AIDE
CODE OF ETHICS

Home Care Aides employed by Plusmore Home Care, Inc. assigned to provide care within a client's home are obligated to conform to the following code of ethics. Please report violations of this code to your supervisor.

Plusmore Employees will NOT:

- Consume the client's food or drink (excluding tap water).
- Discuss his/her own or other's personal problems, religious or political beliefs with the client.
- Use the client's telephone to make or receive personal calls.
- Accept gifts or loans of cash from the client.
- Bring any person, other than another authorized Plusmore Home Care, Inc. employee, to the client's home or disclose to any other person personal information regarding the client or otherwise breach the client's right to privacy and confidentiality of information and records.
- Consume alcoholic beverages in the client's home or during working hours.
- Use drugs for any purpose, other than those medically necessary, at any time.
- Smoke in the client's home.
- Purchase any item from the client, even at fair market value.
- Assume the control of the financial or personal affairs of the client or the client's estate including power of attorney, conservatorship, or guardianship.
- Reside with the client in either the client's or their own home.
- Take or borrow anything from the client or the client's home.
- Use the client's automobile for any reasons, without prior written agreement from both the client and the Program Supervisor.
- Commit any act of abuse, neglect, or exploitation.
- Ask the client to sign a time sheet before the work is completed.

The Home Care Aide shall be allowed to use the bathroom facilities of the client, and with the client's consent, eat a lunch provided by the Home Care Aide.

Figure 3.1. Plusmore Home Care, Inc. Code of Ethics Training Handout (retyped for legibility and to preserve agency anonymity).

edly emphasized the company's strict policy that workers should only ask clients to sign time sheets verifying the worker's hours at the end of each shift, noting that there were serious risks if clients signed for multiple days at once, or at the beginning of the shift, because schedules could change or an emergency could force a worker to leave early. Workers were held liable for any inaccuracies on their time sheets, regardless of circumstance. Inaccuracies could lead to workers being underpaid, or accused of fraud.

At both home care agencies, a large number of formal company rules were intended to circumscribe flows of money, objects, and personal information between older adults and home care workers. Company rules (see figure 3.2) provided to Plusmore employees as part of their

COMPANY RULES

Following are offenses considered serious violations of Company rules. Violation of these rules will result in disciplinary action and/or termination. This list is not all-inclusive and may be amended at any time.

1. Field employees may never solicit and/or purchase items from clients or a client's family, relatives, or associates to provide services of any kind for compensation or otherwise, including services that are not a part of the services provided by the company.

2. Field employees must not stay in the client's home if the client is not present. If the client chooses to leave, explain to the client that if he/she needs to leave for whatever reason, you must also leave. Under no circumstance should you accept or ask a client for a key to the residence.

3. Never borrow money from or lend money to the client.

4. **Do not accept gifts from the clients.** This is for your protection. Some clients have short memories; therefore it is possible that they could give you something one day and forget the next. Also, a family member may notice the item missing and question the client.

5. Do all the assigned tasks to the best of your ability and ONLY THOSE THAT YOU ARE AUTHORIZED TO DO. If the client becomes angry with you for any reason, **do not argue with the client** or raise your voice. Refer the client to your Supervisor. It is your Supervisor's responsibility to handle these problems. It is more important for you to keep a positive working relationship with your client.

6. Employees may not sleep, rest, watch television, or participate in leisure activities while at work.

7. The client's home is your work place. You must respect the client's privacy. You are not to take anyone to a client's home regardless of whether you are asked to or not. This includes children, family members, or friends. Do not discuss your personal or financial problems with the client. Your client most likely has problems also. Do not burden her/him with yours.

8. Never get involved with your client's personal problems, especially when it includes other family members.

9. Never discuss religion or politics with your client or client's family. This could cause hurt feelings and make your job more difficult to do.

10. Clients are **only** transported by automobile with the Supervisor's permission. In areas where using a client's car is required, do not use a client's car unless you have been authorized by your supervisor. In these cases, the client must sign a release and provide a current certificate of insurance for the automobile.

11. Smoking is not allowed while working. Even if your client smokes, you are not permitted to smoke.

Figure 3.2. Plusmore Home Care, Inc. Company Rules. (retyped for legibility and to preserve company anonymity. Font emphases reproduced from original).

12. Phone calls: No personal calls should be made from the client's home. You may call the office, but please ask the client for permission before doing so. Most clients are on limited incomes, so only make the necessary calls that are permitted. The employee will be responsible for payment of unauthorized phone calls, and disciplinary action will be taken for improper use of the client's telephone.

13. Employees may not eat or drink client's food or beverages.

General Instructions

1. Do not wear valuable or cumbersome jewelry, such as big rings and dangling bracelets. You will have to remove these items while cleaning or doing personal care, and therefore, you are taking a chance of losing them.

2. Do not carry a large bag to work with you. Neighbors may be suspicious and may assume you are taking things from the client's home.

3. Remember, your clients may be hard of hearing. Instead of yelling, it is best to face your client and speak slowly.

4. If your client is blind, it is important to remember not to move things around. For example, when you clean the countertop, put things back where you found them. Be aware of this when cleaning every room. This is very important to the client's well being.

5. Dress Code: Wear clean clothing that is comfortable, such as a smock and slacks. Wear flat shoes or athletic shoes with rubber soles. Do not wear open toe shoes or sandals, faded/ripped jeans, halter tops, or shorts. In some areas a uniform may be required. Some operations may have more specific dress code requirements. Always wear your ID badge.

6. Employees should carry a street map.

Confidentiality

The Company acknowledges legal and ethical responsibility to protect the right to privacy of clients and employees. Consequently, the indiscriminate or unauthorized review, use, or disclosure of any personal information regarding any client or employee is expressly prohibited except when required in the regular course of business. Any violation of this policy shall constitute grounds for severe disciplinary action, including possible termination of the offending employee.

Financial and Personal Involvement

You are never to put yourself on a joint checking account with the client, assume power of attorney, be designated as a substitute payee, or be named as beneficiary in the client's estate. You must never be involved in any of the above mentioned situations with any member of the household.

training materials described these restrictions as ways of protecting workers and older adults from becoming enmeshed in complex webs of interdependence that might harm either or both of them. Some of the rules circumscribed the boundaries of workers' labor by prohibiting them from performing unauthorized tasks. The company rules also explain that workers should avoid accepting gifts from clients for their "protection. Some clients have short memories, therefore it is possible they could give you something one day and forget the next." Though the video the workers watched earlier in the morning encouraged flows of care, concern, and personal involvement from workers to older adults, the rules attempted to prevent flows of concern or material items from moving in the reverse direction. As Alicia explained the agency code of ethics, she emphasized that these rules were meant to prevent complicated entanglements. Such entanglements could create burdens for vulnerable older adults or subject workers to expectations beyond those for which they were paid. Despite these rules, over time workers and older adults often build relationships of solidarity and mutuality through illicit exchanges, with workers completing tasks that exceeded clients' formal care plans and older adults reciprocating with favors and gifts.[9]

The first day of training at Plusmore exposed prospective home care workers to several of the central tensions that arise as home care is made into paid work. On the one hand, care is expected to involve close personal relationships, even forms of love. But workers are not supposed to share personal information with their clients. Care workers are expected to view the families of those for whom they care as team mates, but workers should not take sides in family arguments. Care workers should not be in it for the money, yet they should also submit to the management of a hierarchical organization profiting from their labor. These contradictions and tensions reflect the complex role agencies play in mediating between the various rules and norms at play in paid home care work. In this case, care worker training reproduces ideologies of care as private, personal, and motivated by affect rather than material need. The norms and rules conveyed in training simultaneously attempt to curtail potentially messy, interdependent flows of affect, material assistance, and control that emerge in part as a result of these ideologies of care. Instead, worker training reimagined and generated care as work involving unidirectional flows of affect and assistance from workers to clients, with only wages flowing back to workers.

Determining Need

The initial contact between older adults seeking publicly funded services and the Illinois CCP focused on the fair and efficient distribution of taxpayer-funded resources. Before older adults could be referred to service providers like Plusmore, a case manager (employed by another state-contracted service provider) evaluated their eligibility for state-funded services. CCP case managers typically conducted these assessments at older adults' homes. To be deemed eligible, older adults had to provide documentation that they were over the age of 60, residents of Illinois, and US citizens. Each CCP applicant also had to prove that they owned assets totaling less than $17,500, not including their home, car, personal furniture, burial insurance, and several other forms of exempt assets.[10] Finally, case managers used a standardized form called the Determination of Need (DON; see figure 3.3) to assess whether the applicant had the requisite amount of unmet need for care to qualify for program services. Clients' unique lifestyles and preferences played little role in their initial interactions with the CCP. This process contrasted sharply with the individually attuned and affectively warm care promoted by the video shown to Plusmore workers on their first day of training.

The CCP program receives funding from Medicaid waiver programs, which are meant to provide care to those who might otherwise be institutionalized. CCP eligibility standards therefore stipulate that clients require a level of care that would necessitate institutionalization if such needs could not be met at home. CCP case managers determined the amount and type of services necessary to maintain older adults in their homes using the DON form. The DON enumerates criteria to systematically evaluate the kind and degree of older adults' physical and cognitive disabilities, transforming these evaluations into a numerical DON score. The score is based on a widely used measure of cognitive ability called the Mini-Mental State Exam, and a standard list of "Activities of Daily Living and Instrumental Activities of Daily Living" (ADLs and IADLs) widely used to assess the capacities of disabled and older people. These

III. BEHAVIORAL HEALTH (CONTINUED): MINI-MENTAL STATE EXAMINATION

Case manager is to administer all 11 questions equivalent to a score of 30.

_____ (5) 1. What is the (year) (season) (date) (day) (month)?

_____ (5) 2. Where are we: (state) (county) (town) (nursing facility/hospital) (floor)?

_____ (3) 3. Name 3 objects. Allow 1 second to say each. Ask the client all 3 after you have said them. Give 1 point for each CORRECT answer in the first trial only. Then repeat the 3 objects until the client learns all 3. Count trials and repeat the 3 objects until the client learns all 3. Count trials and record. Trials _____

_____ (5) 4. Spell "WORLD" backwards. Score 1 point for each letter in the CORRECT order.

_____ "D" _____ "L" _____ "R" _____ "O" _____ "W"

_____ (3) 5. Ask for the 3 objects repeated in question 3. Give 1 point for each CORRECT answer.

_____ (2) 6. Identify a pencil and a watch.

_____ (1) 7. Repeat the following: "No ifs, ands or buts."

_____ (3) 8. Follow a 3-stage command: "Take a paper in your right hand, fold it in half and put it in your lap."

_____ (1) 9. Read and obey the following: CLOSE YOUR EYES.

_____ (1) 10. Write a sentence.

_____ (1) 11. Copy a design.

Maximum score is 30. Enter **TOTAL** correct answers for MMSE score. → → →

1. For MMSE box below: If score is equal or more than "21"—enter "0"; if score is "20" or less—enter "10"

2. For the MMSE Plus score: Add an additional 10 points to the total MMSE Box below, if appropriate documentation is provided for all three listed below. (Rule 240:715, d) 1) C))

Court adjudication as incompetent or disabled; Physician/Psychiatrist certifies need for 24 hour supervision; **and,** Physician/Psychiatrist certifies presence of Alzheimer's disease, OBS, or dementia.

A **NON-COGNITIVE PROBLEM** is affecting the MMSE score: ☐ **YES** ☐**NO** If yes, **check the correct non-cognitive problem below:**

☐ **Vision/Hearing Problem** ☐ **Language Barrier** ☐ **Low Education/Can't Read** ☐ **Physical Impairment** ☐ **Other:**

If Mini-Mental State Examination score total is: 21–30, proceed with the DON; informant not needed. 20 points or less: An informant may be needed.

1. Informant Available: Y or N **2. Informant Used:** Y or N **3. Name:** _____ **4. Relationship:** _____

Figure 3.3a. CCP Determination of Need Form. Cognitive assessment: Mini-Mental State Examination (top half of form, continues in figure 3.3b).

DETERMINATION OF NEED (Functional Status -- Activities of Daily Living/Instrumental Activities of Daily Living)

FUNCTION	A. LEVEL OF IMPAIRMENT				B. UNMET NEED FOR CARE				Service by CCP	Service by Other	FREQUENCY - for specific needs only	Notes:
1. Eating	0	1	2	3	0	1	2	3				
2. Bathing	0	1	2	3	0	1	2	3				
3. Grooming	0	1	2	3	0	1	2	3				
4. Dressing	0	1	2	3	0	1	2	3				
5. Transferring	0	1	2	3	0	1	2	3				
6. Continence	0	1	2	3	0	1	2	3				
7. Managing Money	0	1	2	3	0	1	2	3				
8. Telephoning	0	1	2	3	0	1	2	3				
9. Preparing Meals	0	1	2	3	0	1	2	3				
10. Laundry	0	1	2	3	0	1	2	3				
11. Housework	0	1	2	3	0	1	2	3				
12. Outside Home	0	1	2	3	0	1	2	3				
13. Routine Health	0	1	2	3	0	1	2	3				
14. Special Health	0	1	2	3	0	1	2	3				
15. Being Alone	0	1	2	3	0	1	2	3				
TOTAL	0				0							

MMSE	A	MMSE/A TOTAL	B	TOTAL DON SCORE
	0	0		

IL-402-1230 (Rev 3/08)

Version 2.0

Figure 3.3b. CCP Determination of Need Form. ADL/IADL assessment (bottom half of form, continues from figure 3.3a).

include a range of tasks understood as necessary for everyday functioning and health, ranging from "eating" and "continence" to "managing money" and "housework." For each activity, the DON also assigns a numerical score corresponding to the individual's "unmet need for assistance" indicating whether an individual received regular help from a "non-CCP resource in the community (e.g., friends, family, local services)." Higher DON scores qualified older adults for larger allocations of funding which translated into a greater number of hours of service paid for by the CCP.

The DON is also used to generate each client's specific service plans, also called "care plans." These care plans typically list the activities for which the client has been authorized to receive assistance from a care worker. Notably, the DON awarded the same number of points (which translated to dollars) for qualitatively different activities, meaning that the amount of care hours a client was allocated did not necessarily correspond to the time needed to accomplish the needed activities. For example, preparing a meal could easily take an hour, while helping a client transfer from bed to chair might only take five minutes. It was the responsibility of Plusmore supervisors to figure out how to best meet clients' preferences within these restrictive, bureaucratically determined care plans.

The Determination of Need tool represents one way that public moral logics about fairness and equitable access to public resources remake older adults and their households in the context of home care services. Information studies scholar Bernd Frohmann argues that, particularly in service industries, "the construction, hence the *being*, of the service depends on its descriptions." The DON generates a universalizing definition of care by classifying diverse ways of living into equivalent and generic "activities of daily life." This bureaucratic practice intentionally considers older adults' broader social relations in a narrow and transactional manner, focusing only on the assistance these relations provide. In the process, the DON reduces the rich tapestry of older adults' daily lives and histories to generic descriptions of incapacity and need, and then transforms these needs into abstractions: a numerical DON score and a corresponding dollar figure.

The DON designates particular tasks as the realm of care and particular individuals as subjects in need of care. The DON, much like other bureaucratic documents, generates specific types of subjects and regimes of control. Anthropologist Matthew Hull describes bureaucratic documents as having the "generative capacity" to construct things, subjects, forms of sociality, and regimes of control. In particular, Hull argues that documents mediate between schemes of classification and particular people, places, and things, constructing "*this* person as a victim or *this* house as an encroachment."[11] With paid home care, the DON classifies some kinds of people as deserving of public assistance: those who are old, have limited assets, and limited ability to meet their daily needs. The DON generates older adults as needy subjects on the basis of individual incapacities and individual resources. The form draws a boundary between the client and the rest of their household; family members are taken in to account only to the extent that they make claims on assets or help older adults accomplish daily activities. Older adults' other emotional and social capacities, as well as their contributions to family and community, have limited relevance to the DON. By evaluating older adults apart from their broader social contexts, the DON instantiates them as individual subjects of equitable and fair bureaucratic regimes of control.

By enacting ideologies of individualism, the DON establishes the state as an ethical arbiter of resource distribution. The DON produced a relatively impersonal and seemingly fair process through which to compare the needs of diverse older adults and then allocate the limited resources available to the Community Care Program in accordance with broader program and legislative goals. This was not an unintentional by-product of bureaucratic management, but its goal. Though individual case managers could interpret and manipulate the DON form to reflect their judgment about individual adults, use of the DON produced significant limits on the extent to which discretion, favoritism, or discrimination might influence the allocation of public resources. Thus, the DON assessment tool was intended not only to be objective, but also to objectify older adults in order to ensure the equal rights and access of all of Illinois's citizens and legal residents over the age of 60 to publicly funded social services.[12] In this sense, assessment tools like the DON are central to the functioning of a democratic welfare state because of (rather than despite) their abstracting and objectifying tendencies.[13]

Though most older adults understand good care as deeply responsive to their particular preferences and social relations, the DON allocates care on the basis of needs that the state pre-determines as objective and universal. This is one reason publicly funded care is often described as impersonal and inferior to privately funded care. Supervisors at publicly funded home care agencies are tasked with mediating between these conflicting understandings of care.

Enacting Care Plans

Plusmore supervisors' labor was ethically complex, requiring them to reconcile abstract, homogenizing rules and legal regulations with the messy and particular lives of their workers and clients.[14] One of the reasons older adults wish to remain in their homes is because they can continue to exercise the rights of private property that enable them to be seen as independent persons. Yet, when home care workers entered elders' homes, so too did a variety of government laws, agency rules, and market pressures that had to be negotiated alongside older adults' preferences. Most of these laws were developed with non-domestic workplaces in mind, and sometimes conflicted with the domestic norms and prerogatives of older adults' households. For example, equal opportunity laws prohibit employers from discriminating on the basis of race, gender, age, and other protected categories. Yet individuals typically retain the right to use any criteria they choose when deciding who may enter their homes. Health and safety laws prohibit workers from activities likely to cause injury, like lifting heavy objects or climbing on ladders. Yet such activities are common to household tasks with which older adults expect assistance. Supervisors were charged with implementing care plans in ways that simultaneously upheld laws and respected older adults' preferences and needs.

Plusmore supervisors first interacted with new clients after case managers faxed the agency their care plans. These documents listed the number of service hours the client had been allocated each month and the ADLs and IADLS with which the client needed assistance. Upon receiving a new client's care plan, the supervisor in charge of the region of the city in which the client lived would open electronic and paper files for the new case and call the new client. Because of their large caseloads,

Plusmore supervisors were only able to contact clients by telephone. Their initial conversations with new clients were typically fraught with tension, as supervisors tried to align the client's direct requests with their care plan and with the schedules and skills of available care workers.

One summer afternoon, Plusmore supervisor Ruby Watkins received a care plan for a client approved for 15 hours of service per week, to start as soon as possible. As soon as she received the fax, Ruby started looking through her list of workers. She noted which workers had told her they wanted more hours of work and which were working less than 25 hours. The agency could not afford the time-and-a-half overtime pay if she assigned someone more than 40 total hours. She identified two workers with availability in the afternoons, which she hoped would work for the client.

With a plan in mind, Ruby dialed the client's number. When the client's daughter answered the phone, Ruby launched into a well-practiced description of Plusmore's services and her role. The daughter, impatient, told Ruby that she needed help bathing her bed-bound mother and turning her over. Ruby explained that because of government health and safety regulations, Plusmore workers were not allowed to lift anything heavier than 15 pounds. Lifting or turning the client might be a problem. In these cases, clients often needed to have an expensive piece of equipment installed in the home to assist with lifting. Insurance or Medicare might help pay for it, but it would require some time-consuming bureaucratic wrangling. The daughter assured Ruby that the worker could just assist her with baths and turns, and would not be performing these tasks alone.

The daughter agreed to have a worker come in the afternoon, as long as Ruby promised not to "just send me some girl." Upon hearing the word "girl," Ruby became concerned. She quickly responded that "we can't discriminate by age, but the two people I have in mind for you are grown. One is 49 and has been with the company for three years, the other is 53 and has been with the company for over 20 years. Both are very good." Many of Plusmore's clients were disinclined toward younger workers, believing them to be inexperienced and unreliable. Across agencies, clients' preferences for and prejudices against particular kinds of workers frequently ran afoul of national moral commitments to equal opportunity. These conflicts pit the nation's egalitarian ethics against laws that protect inhabitants' rights to control what happens on private property. Though Ruby acknowledged and accommodated the daughter's preferences, she was compelled to emphasize the agency's adherence both to worker safety regulations and equal employment statutes. In the process, she signaled to the client that individual preferences could only be accommodated to the extent they did not conflict with labor protections.

Plusmore management placed a premium on making sure that the company provided every possible hour of care assigned to its clients by the CCP because of its slim profit margins. Its shareholders' earnings were generated through the economies of scale created by providing tens of thousands of hours of care each month. Agency incentive structures rewarded supervisors for the number of filled "service hours" as a primary measure of successful care. Supervisors received bonuses if they were able to provide at least 87 percent of the service hours allocated to their clients each month. In focusing on the provision of service hours, Plusmore policies simultaneously neglect alternative criteria for assessing care, such as the quality and duration of care relationships, or care workers' attunement to clients' ways of life. Prioritizing service hour delivery meant treating care workers as interchangeable laborers, such that any worker was considered fit to care for any client. By incentivizing this quantitative measure of managerial success, Plusmore policy imagined home care workers and older adults as abstract independent individuals rather than as persons with unique histories enmeshed in complex social relations.

Supervisors were left to discern how to deliver service hours to actual in-the-flesh people. Keeping service levels high was challenging. Clients sometimes canceled service hours because they had a doctor's appointment or family event. Workers periodically needed a day off because they were sick or had family obligations. Service hour totals were calculated weekly. If supervisors were made aware of schedule changes quickly, they could often make up missed hours by altering the schedule or offering a substitute worker. Supervisors were typically lenient with workers who needed to take a day off if the worker provided sufficient notice for the supervisor to assign a substitute. Plusmore did not offer paid sick or family leave, but workers would not lose their jobs for missing a day of work. Plusmore was able to accommodate these absences because it kept a stable of "perm-temp" workers available as substitutes.[15] However, some older adults were reluctant to allow strange substitute workers into their homes. Supervisors typically removed workers from their cases if they failed to provide adequate notice of an absence that caused the agency to lose service hour reimbursements more than once.[16]

In the process of translating care plans into everyday care, Plusmore supervisors navigated between intentionally abstract bureaucratic and legal mandates and the dynamic complexity of clients' and workers' actual lives and needs. Plusmore supervisors consistently expressed a strong ethic of fairness, working to balance the preferences of clients with the rights and needs of their employees. They did so working within an organization that rewarded them for filling service hours, but did not have clear mechanisms for monitoring or rewarding the complex ethical labor that filled their workdays.

"She's Not There to Take Care of the Whole Family"

CCP care plans determine older adults' needs as independent individuals, rather than as persons embedded in complex webs of care. Plusmore clients frequently lived with family members, leaving supervisors to disentangle the generative labor required to sustain elders from that required to sustain their households. Imagining elders as independent from their households was a useful fiction that made it possible for the state to fund care for vulnerable older adults without being accused of paying for poor families' housekeepers. Within households, workers often struggled to enact boundaries as clear as those imagined by care plans and agency policy. Supervisors frequently mediated the conflicts that arose when older adults' care could not be so easily separated from care of their households.

One afternoon, I sat in Jackie Wilson's cubicle at the Plusmore office as she attempted to resolve a "headache" of a case. Problems started when a client's son kicked the worker out of the home he shared with his mother, telling her not to return. According to the worker, the son insisted that she was responsible for various household tasks that were not included on his mother's care plan. The son wanted the worker to clean up after the dog, wash all the household's dishes, and clean the entire house. Jackie told the worker to leave the job and not return until Jackie called her back. Jackie recorded the day as a "lock out" on the worker's time sheet so that the worker (and the agency) would be paid for a complete shift even though the client had not signed her time sheet for that day's work.

As we sat together, Jackie called the client's son. Jackie calmly told the son that she had heard he was having a problem with his mother's home care worker. She suggested that they review his mother's care plan again to make sure that everyone was on the same page. Without giving the son time to interject, Jackie began reviewing the restrictions on what the care worker was allowed to do in the client's home. She emphasized that such limitations were imposed by the service needs delineated by the DON and by agency policies meant to protect the health and safety of their workers. "The home care aide is only supposed to take care of the client, even though other people lived there with her. She can wash your mom's dishes and make her bed. She can clean your mom's commode, the bathroom sink, your mom's bedroom and the area around mom's chair in the bedroom. She can't wash the whole family's dishes; she can't clean up after the dog. She can't scrub the toilet; she can't scrub the bathtub except after she's given your mom a bath or clean other areas of the house that your mom doesn't use. She's not there to clean up after the whole family, just mom." Jackie told me later that the son had argued that he sometimes left a pot in the sink, but not a week's worth of dishes. He did not understand why the worker could not wash one more pot. Jackie repeated her description of the client's care plan. She later told me she was hoping that by repeating the plan several times, the son would start to remember it. Instead, the son interrupted again and said that if there was an extra pot in the sink, he didn't understand why it would be against the rules for the home care worker to wash it if he cooked his mom's meal in it. Rather than responding to the son's objections, Jackie told him she would send a quality assurance (QA) supervisor to the house with a new home care worker on Monday. The QA supervisor would show the worker and the son how the care plan applied to their household.[17]

A little while later, the phone rang again. The son wanted to know if his mother's home care worker would still be paid for days when she didn't show up for work. Jackie responded that she was confused, since the son never mentioned that the worker had missed her appointments. Suspicious about the veracity of this claim, Jackie told the son that he had signed the worker's time sheets verifying that the worker had been present. Therefore, Plusmore was legally required to pay the care worker for those hours. Jackie spoke bluntly: if the son had a problem with a worker not showing up consistently, he should call her immediately and not bundle his concerns with other accusations.

Workers were summarily fired when the agency could prove that clients signed time sheets for unworked days. The agency considered this "time sheet fraud," a form of theft from both the agency and the state. In this case, however, Jackie was concerned that the son's accusation was a case of unfulfilled expectations. She suspected that the client's son had signed the worker's time sheet for days the worker was absent, essentially giving the worker paid days off. He probably expected that the worker would reciprocate this gift by doing extra housework not listed in the care plan. When the worker refused to complete the additional tasks, Jackie guessed the son had grown irate and kicked her out. Such arrangements were common sources of conflict when workers and clients differently interpreted vague expectations of reciprocity. Without any reliable proof that this is what had occurred, Jackie decided not to fire the care worker, but did give her a harsh warning about the consequences of time sheet fraud.

Plusmore's training video urged workers to consider clients' families as teammates. CCP care plans imagined clients as individuals whose lives could be untangled from their households. This might mean that workers were expected to leave a dirty toilet next to a freshly cleaned sink, or a clear circle around an elders' favored recliner in an otherwise cluttered and dusty living room. Home care agency policies also presumed that workers could provide care to one member of a household without becoming enmeshed in household reciprocities. Yet in many cases, workers were unable to avoid entanglements with clients' kin, which sometimes proved problematic. Plusmore supervisors were left the ethically tricky task of untangling enmeshed relations by articulating boundaries between older adults, their households and kin, and home care workers. Supervisors generate older adults as independent persons by insisting that older adults and their household members should be treated as separate individuals with distinct rights and needs rather than as collectives.

"Whatever It Takes"

Belltower's business depended on attracting and retaining adequate numbers of clients to pay its bills. This included overhead costs, staff compensation, and contributions to the coffers of the larger elder-services organization to which it belonged. Plusmore supervisors were pressured to provide generic, abstract service hours to clients regardless of clients' idiosyncratic situations and personalities. In contrast, Belltower supervisors faced competing pressures to provide the flexible, responsive care that clients desired while keeping their fees reasonable and generating enough revenue to stay in business. Belltower supervisors faced pressure to accommodate clients, even when clients' demands were at odds with government laws or agency policy. Belltower's orientation toward consumer satisfaction shaped supervisors' hiring, marketing, and conflict management practices. Their focus on consumer satisfaction sometimes made it challenging to also protect workers' needs and rights.

Belltower supervisors preferred workers whose moral commitments to care motivated them to do more than required by their official job descriptions. Belltower could only offer near-minimum wages, and struggled to recruit workers who could deliver the flexible care they promised their clients.[18] Supervisors argued that workers with strong moral commitments to care would provide the flexible care clients desired, exceeding the limitations of narrow job descriptions and the labor expected of minimum-wage workers. At the time of my fieldwork, the agency offered no formal training. They thus preferred workers with previous experience caring for older adults. Many Belltower workers had previously worked for publicly funded agencies that provided training, while others had been the primary caregiver for aging parents. Belltower relied on various welfare-to-work programs, word of mouth, and current home care workers' social networks to recruit workers with the necessary moral commitment and skill.

Belltower supervisors sought workers who had been previously socialized into particular understandings of domesticity and care. Such workers typically had been socialized to care by kin, and kin often continued to support and be supported by their labor in multiple ways. For example, Carmen Rodriguez, a Belltower supervisor, referred to her own work, and that of her employees, as "more than a job, it's a mission." She used the notion of care as a mission to describe why she sometimes accepted cases in which older adults' needs exceeded the agency's normal capacity. For example, she assigned a single worker to care for an incontinent, bedridden older man and his mentally disabled son so that their wife/mother could undergo knee replacement surgery. The family lived in a cramped garden apartment and could not afford more than one worker. Carmen took the case, aware of the exceptional amount of labor she was asking of the employee she assigned to the case. She told me that "cases like this are part of our mission. Good caregivers will take these kinds of difficult cases because that's the mission. Some workers only want to take easy cases with rich families who only need cooking and cleaning, but we need to take the ones that need more care." While Carmen described the "need" to take clients who required exceptional amounts of care as part of a moral mission, it was also true that the agency had to recruit clients in a range of circumstances to fund its activities. While Belltower did not train workers to approach their caregiving as a mission, agency supervisors looked for workers inclined toward this approach. Workers were expected to already have a deeply moral attachment to care and see it as more than a route to a paycheck.

Carmen continued, saying "Some Filipina caregivers think they are too good for some kinds of cases, they don't want to change diapers or do sponge baths. I want the caregivers who will do whatever it takes to care for the client, the ones who clearly go above and beyond." Implicit in Carmen's suggestion that workers' cultural backgrounds shape their approaches to care was an understanding that the qualities she most valued in caregivers did not come from their training as care workers. Instead, she suggested that workers were socialized by particular kinds of families and ethnic communities to "do whatever it takes." In this way, Belltower and privately funded agencies like it capitalize on the generative labor of workers' kin and communities. They need workers' families to instill in workers the forms of moral imagination and dedication that make their business possible.

As I watched Belltower supervisors interview and evaluate potential workers, the multiple ways in which the agency depends on others to socialize and train workers became clear. For example, early one morning, Carmen invited me to join her in interviewing Daronda, a potential new hire. Carmen began the interview by asking Daronda to tell us a little about herself. Daronda described herself as "just a single mom trying to make it with no money coming in" since she lost her last job. Throughout the interview Carmen indicated that she did not think Daronda had the requisite moral commitment or aesthetic socialization to care for Belltower clients. Carmen immediately drew my attention to Daronda's attire, whispering to me in a conspiratorial tone, "Did you notice her shoes?" Daronda's outfit was an awkward approximation of American business attire, perhaps all she could manage without steady income. She wore a grey double-breasted pin-stripe suit, with no blouse and the skirt hemmed six inches above her knees. She wore clear plastic high-heeled sandals, and a large blister was visible above the knuckle of her big toe. To Carmen, Daronda's clothing signaled that she did not have the requisite understanding of middle-class tastes to succeed at Belltower. Carmen's first impression of Daronda was driven home later in the interview during a role-playing exercise. Carmen pronounced herself an older, diabetic female client, and asked Daronda to describe what meals she would prepare. Carmen later told me that Daronda's answers suggested she did not have the skills required to cook meals that their clients would find acceptable. The role-play exercise suggests that she was also looking for workers who had the embodied experience to respond to specific requests that reflected specific tastes and preferences.

Carmen and other supervisors scrutinized potential workers' style of dress and cooking as indicators of their caregiving skills. Dress and culinary skill were indicators of workers' abilities to reproduce middle-class aesthetic norms, as interpreted by supervisors. Workers who could adopt the outward signs of sharing middle-class tastes (e.g., cooking the right foods, wearing their clothes in the right ways) were workers with whom Belltower's middle- and upper-class clientele would feel comfortable.[19] Home care workers who show a fluent ability to embody multiple ways of life learn such skills from their friends and family. This is an additional layer of generative labor performed by families and capitalized upon by agencies.[20] Workers' families are implicitly expected to serve as a critical training ground for workers' domestic skills and aesthetics. In the process, diverse forms of domesticity inculcated in workers by their families are subjected to ongoing judgment, with significant economic consequences.

"We Take Care of All That for You"

To maintain an adequate client base, Belltower supervisors constantly marketed the agency and tried to recruit new clients. To stay in business, Belltower competed with other agencies and less expensive forms of care provision. This forced the agency to view older adults as consumers with the power to take their business elsewhere. Agency staff promoted the agency's services by highlighting the ways that supervisors, rather than older adults, would be responsible for handling confusing legal and financial rules and managing any predictable conflicts that arose between workers and clients.

The agency lost clients when they moved to nursing homes, entered the hospital, or died. Each lost client meant one or more workers went without a paycheck until the agency could find another suitable match. Belltower vice president Debra Collins spent a portion of every staff meeting impressing on supervisors the importance of marketing the agency's services to grow the client base and seeking new ideas about how to extend the agency's reach. Supervisors were supposed to spend a portion of their time each week convincing regional professionals who worked with older adults to recommend Belltower's services. Although necessary to sustain the agency's business, supervisors loathed marketing, describing it as awkward "begging." They told me they had been attracted to their jobs to help older adults, not to work as "salespeople."

It was a good day for Belltower supervisors when they received a call from an older adult looking for home care services. Supervisors visited potential clients in their home as soon as possible. Supervisors also described these visits as "marketing visits," which had dual goals: to promote the agency's services and assess the potential client's needs and preferences. As supervisors met with potential clients, they learned what clients expected and feared from home care. During these marketing visits, Belltower supervisors focused on justifying the cost of agency services, emphasizing that the agency would relieve clients of the work of being employers and would provide personalized care. Supervisors typically avoided describing the legal and economic complexities of actually providing services.

My visit to the Schmidt sisters' home with supervisor Kathy Hirschorn was typical of Belltower's marketing home visits. The day before our visit, one sister called Kathy to inquire about hiring the agency to care for the other sister. Kathy did not waste any time, scheduling an appointment to meet the Schmidt sisters as soon as possible. She did not want the family to call another agency before she could convince them to hire Belltower. Kathy did not take it for granted that interested older adults would necessarily become clients; it was her job to convince them.

When we arrived at the Schmidt home, Kathy thanked the sisters for inviting us and quickly launched into an explanation of Belltower's services. She distinguished Belltower from other service providers by describing how the agency would protect the client from the unpleasantness that could come from being an employer. At the same time, she said, Belltower provided clients with the control and flexibility to determine what happened in their own homes. This was in contrast to other methods of finding home care workers, so "even though you might hear from your friends that it is less expensive to use one of those registries, or to hire a worker yourself, make sure you think that through. When you use a registry or hire someone directly, you become their employer, which means you are in charge of everything. Paying payroll taxes. Would you run a background check? What happens if your worker is sick? At Belltower we take care of all that for you." According to Kathy, hiring Belltower meant older adults could have workers in their own homes without becoming subject to the legal demands made on employers or losing the control associated with living in one's own home.

After outlining the benefits of hiring Belltower versus other kinds of providers, Kathy asked why the sisters were interested in hiring a home care worker. As we listened to their story, Kathy asked a series of clarifying questions with a practiced air, taking extensive notes. Throughout the interview, Kathy anticipated and responded to the sisters' anxieties about having a worker intimately involved in their household. She described how Belltower managed home care workers and made sure the new worker blended seamlessly into the rhythms of the household. When the healthier sister expressed concern over her disabled sister's weight loss, Kathy asked about preferred meals. She assured the sisters that she would find a home care worker who could prepare excellent versions of their favorite foods. In response to one sister's concern that the worker be "honest," Kathy reemphasized that Belltower would not employ anyone untrustworthy; that was another benefit of hiring a full-service agency. Kathy emphasized that agency staff interviewed, checked references, and ran criminal background checks for every new employee. In contrast to registry services or hiring someone through word of mouth, at Belltower, she said, "We know our employees, we know what they are good at, so we can find someone who will be a good fit for you."

Toward the end of the interview, Kathy asked what kind of personality would fit best in her household, offering several prompts. After a moment of consideration, the healthier sister noted that the other sister had "the softest touch you'll ever meet." She thought a care worker with a strong work ethic was more important for the sisters' well-being than the workers' relational skills. As the healthier sister put it, "I'm not saying there won't be love and friendship and all that, but it's bad if the person doesn't do her work and creates stress." The ideal home care worker would be someone who could get instructions at the beginning of the day and just figure out what needed to be done. Her sister couldn't handle a worker who was "lazy and needs to be bossed." Kathy responded that this was another reason to hire Belltower. With the agency's involvement, she said, neither sister would have to confront a worker in the unlikely event that there were problems. They could just call a supervisor who would fix the problem. Kathy's pitch persuasively framed Belltower as relieving the sisters of all the responsibilities of an employer, while also providing care attuned to their unique tastes.

In marketing its services, Belltower set few hard limits about which services it would provide, except for those prohibited by health and safety regulations. Kathy suggested that this ethic stemmed from the agency's non-profit and faith-based status. She maintained that "service is at the heart of what we do. When someone does not have a family, we try to fill that role and bring care to the situation. We try to stay flexible." Though her language differed from Carmen's emphasis on care as a "mission," both supervisors emphasized the moral aspects of their work. She saw the agency as taking on the roles of absent kin. Imagining care in this way meant that Belltower supervisors imposed relatively few limits on what workers could do. Kathy recognized that the agency had to market its services to clients in order to survive, but did not imagine herself selling a generic commodity. In contrast to Plusmore, which was required to provide care that had been allocated according to the same criteria for each client, Belltower supervisors emphasized how carefully they tailored the care provided to each older adult. Older adults were able to avoid the objectifying, alienating potential of paid care when they had the resources to pay for private care purchased in a free market.

Matchmaking

Throughout Kathy's marketing pitch to the Schmidt sisters, she emphasized that the agency and its staff would be able to provide a worker with a complementary personality, skill set, and cooking repertoire. As soon as we returned to the office, Kathy and Celia Tomas, another supervisor, began talking about which of their care work staff was available for the days that the Schmidt sisters preferred. Finding just the right match was always a challenge. Several Belltower supervisors described this part of their job as "like running a dating service." Being able to find a good match for each client meant maintaining a large and diverse staff to accommodate the wide variety of client preferences and personalities. As matchmakers, supervisors also needed detailed knowledge of their staff members' strengths and skills.

Belltower supervisors' comparison of their work pairing workers and clients with romantic matchmaking illustrated the ways they understood their work as providing private, familial forms of intimacy and care to their clients. Yet the matchmaking metaphor was limited because supervisors were focused primarily on meeting the desires of only one partner: the client. Unlike romantic matchmakers, home care supervisors were also responsible for upholding a number of federal statutes that governed home care as a form of labor, rather than as a form of private intimacy. Supervisors thus had to find ways to meet clients' desires when they conflicted with federal labor and anti-discrimination statutes. In the process, supervisors safeguarded clients' status as private persons and their ability to exercise the liberties of consumer choice.

One of the contradictions supervisors found most troubling was that between protecting clients' prerogatives to allow or deny others entry to their private homes and implementing federal equal employment mandates. A significant minority of Belltower's clients expressed racially discriminatory preferences. Some clients refused workers on the basis of race or nationality. Others expressed strong preferences for non-white women based on racial/cultural stereotypes that women of color would be more nurturing and respectful of elders. Potential clients typically made their preferences known through subtle means during marketing home visits. They might ask specifically for someone who knew how to cook German or Italian food, or use their poor hearing as a reason to request a worker who spoke English "without an accent." Supervisors told me that they personally found these racist requests abhorrent. At the same time, they believed that older adults had the right to refuse anyone entry into their homes, and so there was little they could do to prevent clients from being discriminatory. Supervisors also told me that it was their responsibility as employers to protect their home care workers from working in homes where they might face discrimination. They felt it was to everyone's benefit to accommodate clients' racial preferences. The agency was able to hire workers of all backgrounds and satisfy equal employment statutes because clients were diverse in their bigotry.

I only witnessed one occasion in which a Belltower supervisor refused to provide service to a potential client. The way agency staff navigated this case illuminates the limits of the agency's ability to accommodate clients' discriminatory preferences. Jennifer Martin and I were driving to a home visit in one of Chicago's near-northern suburbs when she received a call from Lena Harris. Jennifer was the director of Belltower Home Care's suburban office, and Lena, one of the agency's supervisors, worked directly under her. Lena would not call while Jennifer was out doing home visits unless the matter was urgent, so Jennifer pulled over and answered her call. Lena, speaking calmly, told Jennifer that she was calling for instructions about how to respond to a potential client who was interested in purchasing at least 40 hours of care per week. Such clients were highly coveted. The potential client told Lena outright that she did not want a black worker coming to her home. From Lena's speech, the client deduced that Lena was black, and asked for another supervisor to come to her home to do the initial interview.

Jennifer was furious. She told Lena that she would handle the situation and that Lena should not worry about it. Jennifer told me that outright bigotry such as this was unusual; she had never before encountered a client so boldly racist as to refuse a visit from a black supervisor. The potential client put Jennifer in a troubling legal position. Jennifer explained that it was one thing for the agency to match workers and older adults based on elders' preferences, but it was something else entirely when an elder's bigotry made it impossible for a supervisor to do her job. While home care workers might be interchanged to meet client demands, Lena's higher position in the organizational hierarchy made such substitutions impossible. Acceding to this demand would be a threat to Lena's employment, and therefor a threat to the agency's compliance with the law. No matter how wealthy the client, how big of a bonanza for the agency's bottom line, or how many workers' jobs would be more secure, it was not possible to serve her and at the same time uphold both Jennifer's and Belltower's legal and moral obligations. As we sat in the car, Jennifer took several deep breaths and called the potential client, telling her that Belltower would be unable to meet her needs. She warned the client that no full-employment home care agency would be able to serve her without violating equal employment laws. She suggested that the client might consider hiring a worker directly or use a registry service. This recommendation signaled the depth of Jennifer's anger, since Belltower supervisors usually did everything possible to discourage clients from directly employing workers and using registry services.

In responding to the preferences of racist clients, Belltower supervisors found themselves straddling the competing demands of two of the United States' most potent laws and values. On the one hand, Belltower was obligated to abide by federal and state equal employment statutes prohibiting employment discrimination. On the other hand, in the United States, individuals have the right to deny whomever they choose entry into their private homes. Mediating between these public and private versions of morality was a constant challenge for supervisors. In order to attract and satisfy as many clients as possible, Belltower supervisors creatively reconciled national and personal egalitarian ethics with the racist demands of their well-to-do clientele, turning this kind of ethical tinkering around race into economic value.

In these initial encounters, Belltower staff treated older adults as consumers with the power to take their business elsewhere. In contrast to the bureaucratic individual subjects generated by publicly funded care practices, privately funded agencies catered to their clients' desires for personalized care. By positioning the agency as an employer protecting older adult consumers from the moral and legal demands of public workplaces, Belltower fostered ideological distinctions between public and private. Supervisors promoted the agency's services as a way of enabling older adults to purchase domestic services in the marketplace while maintaining their homes as private domestic spaces rather than workplaces. This enabled older adults to retain the privileges of independence and consumer freedom in a system built on the privileges of private property.

"Like Sisters"

One of Belltower supervisors' most complex roles was managing the flows of reciprocities and drawing boundaries between care-for-kin and care-for-work in their employees' lives. Even as supervisors described worker-client pairings in intimate terms, they attempted to interrupt the forms of intimacy and obligation that often grew between workers and clients. Unlike at Plusmore, where supervisors could insist on boundaries to which their clients objected, at Belltower, supervisors had to find ways of managing relations while still satisfying their clients' desires.

Belltower supervisor Celia Tomas seemed to spend the entire day, every day, on the phone. She called home care workers, cajoling and pleading with them to take a new case, a few more hours, a difficult client. She answered and returned calls from clients, soothing their anxieties, empathizing with their complaints. Celia's goal was to keep everyone happy. To keep everyone happy while still earning the agency money, Celia and other supervisors depended on the ideologies of care and kinship that workers learned among kin.

Celia's office was small and brightly lit. Only work safety notices, procedural lists, and more than a dozen photocopied calendars of the current month interrupted the white walls. Each calendar represented a different client receiving live-in care from Belltower workers. In each day's box, Celia had written the name of the worker staffing the case. Some boxes had names crossed out and replaced multiple times as schedules and clients' preferences changed. She viewed calendars with multiple changes as messy. They signaled situations where the agency was struggling to provide its customer with the stable, trouble-free, personalized care it promised. Celia also kept a list next to her computer of clients who were receiving care only a few days a week. These were easier to keep track of and did not need their own calendar.

Most mornings during my fieldwork at Belltower's offices, I sat with Celia, observing her on the phone and talking with her about the calls she found interesting. One of these mornings, Celia received a phone call from one of the agency's longest-standing clients. Mr. and Mrs. Trotter, a married couple, received live-in care seven days a week. In order to provide this service without incurring the extra expense of overtime pay, Belltower's policy was to have a "main" worker provide four days of care and a "relief" worker provide three days of care.[21] Despite this significant amount of care, their calendar showed few if any corrections each month—Celia had found stable, well-matched workers for both shifts. Both husband and wife were in their mid-nineties. Mrs. Trotter was experiencing moderately advanced Alzheimer's disease. Mr. Trotter had mild dementia and difficulty walking. Mrs. Trotter was born and raised in East Asia, while Mr. Trotter was born and raised in the United States.[22] The couple continued to participate in a large and active support network, at the center of which was a younger male neighbor with whom they had been close for many years.

That morning, Mr. Trotter called to tell Celia he wanted to stop receiving service on the weekends. Celia was surprised and concerned. The Trotters did not have anyone in their support system who could provide the round-the-clock assistance they needed on the weekends. If they reduced service, the agency would lose a substantial and previously stable revenue stream. She eventually determined that Mr. Trotter was angry that the weekend worker, Constance, had been serving them reheated rice, something his wife would have been furious about earlier in life. He interpreted it as a sign of the worker's laziness. Celia, suspecting a more complicated story, persuaded Mr. Trotter to give Constance one more chance.

After the call, Celia told me that she suspected that the primary care worker, Joramae, might be trying to sabotage the relief worker. Celia had suspected Joramae of sabotage once before. Celia's suspicion was confirmed when Constance reported that Joramae had told her it was okay to serve reheated rice. Celia next called Joramae to chastise her. Clearly frustrated, Celia told Joramae, "We are workers, they are the employers. We are like family." Celia spoke loudly into the phone, instructing Joramae that if she had a problem or concern about one of her colleagues, she should call Celia to discuss it, rather than telling their clients. "From our point of view," Celia said, "this hurts you and the other caregiver. You and she are like sisters and we don't want you badmouthing your other sister. So if you have a problem with your reliever, call us. We have to stick together . . . a minus for the relief worker is a minus for the whole company, so tell us about it because it makes the company look bad." Celia called upon forms of solidarity and support normatively found among kin, insisting the worker display similar loyalty to her co-worker and to the agency.

Though Celia pushed care workers to develop kinships with their colleagues, it was more common that home care workers' relationships with elderly clients reflected their kinship experiences. It was not entirely surprising, then, that Joramae had become involved with the family beyond strict bounds of her employment. Joramae told her she had been planning to visit the Trotters that weekend to cook for their friend's birthday. This confirmed Celia's suspicion that Joramae had sabotaged her colleague so that she could work extra hours for the client. Celia warned Joramae that she would be fired the next time she tried a similar stunt. Celia did not object to care workers providing care to clients' family and friends. Belltower was happy to provide care to clients' extended networks if the clients could pay for it. This contrasted sharply with the rules limiting care to other members of Plusmore clients' households. However, it was problematic when Belltower workers' sense of obligation to their clients or their own households undermined their sense of obligation to the agency and its employees.

From Celia's perspective, Joramae had capitalized on the intimate trusting relationship with a client, inserting herself into the Trotter's familial circuits of care and material reciprocity. Each worker spent hundreds of hours with the Trotters each month, becoming embedded in their clients' daily lives. Celia tried to rework the moral obligations and circuits of reciprocity that often grew between workers and clients by constructing the agency and its employees as family. By arguing that home care workers should consider themselves like sisters, Celia pushed against the forms of solidarity and loyalty that sometimes grew between clients and their home care workers. She suggested that agency employees should feel solidarity and loyalty with one another and understand themselves as structurally opposed to their clients. Her statements promoted a moral separation between persons bound together through care

practices, producing older adults as independent both of the public obligations of employers and of reciprocal kin-like obligations to workers.
Notably excluded from the kinship imaginaries Celia promoted were the
circuits connecting home care workers with their own kin. In managing conflicts, Belltower supervisors demanded that workers transfer the
forms of moral obligation learned from kin to the agency and its clients.

The Moral Labor of Making Care Work

As home care agency staff go about their daily labor of hiring and training workers, recruiting clients, staffing cases, and managing conflicts,
they simultaneously transform care practices into care work. This process
involves embedding everyday care practices within the broader structures of American labor and political economy. For example, everyday
care practices are transformed as rationalized needs assessments turn
daily tasks into numerical scores that are used to allocate public dollars to
purchase services from for-profit corporations. The domestic skills and
ethics that many workers learn among kin are transformed into resources
that agencies depend on to provide flexible, empathic care.

As care practices are transformed into care work, older adults and
workers are treated as though they are separate from broader social and
kin relations. Agency policies and management practices promote particular understandings of both personhood and social relations in paid
care. In publicly funded agencies like Plusmore, older adults are treated
as independent persons whose needs are distinct from those of their
broader social relations. In privately funded agencies like Belltower,
older adults are treated as consumers with the economic independence
to freely choose their service providers. The state's bureaucratic systems
of managing care emphasize the fair distribution of resources, while
consumer-driven models of private care emphasize customer satisfaction. These different ways of managing care have different consequences
for workers. In bureaucratic systems of care, workers are similarly
treated as individuals whose rights must also be maintained according
to standards of equity and fairness. In consumer-driven models of care,
workers' tastes, attributes, and actions are evaluated in terms of how
they support client and agency needs. These different ways of articulating the independence of older adults emphasize different aspects of lib-

eral personhood and different ways of navigating the moral challenges and contradictions that arise in daily care.

Home care agency management practices illustrate the ways that morality becomes indispensable to capitalist economic orders. As home care agency staff go about the business of care, they face a variety of competing pressures to implement the egalitarian ethics encoded in public employment policies, protect the privacy and self-determination of elderly clients, and ensure the economic viability of their agencies. Supervisors face complex ethical dilemmas repeatedly each day, exercising significant discretion interpreting these competing policies. As supervisors negotiate the multiple, often-conflicting values of older adults, families, workers, and the nation in which they live, they not only creatively engage in moral relations, they also justify the existence of the agencies that employ them. In so doing, they render economic value from moral values.

Home care agencies capitalize on workers' experiences of kinship and care. Agency staff hope workers will build close relationships with clients. At the same time, agencies expect that workers will always put their clients' needs before their own, resisting invitations to become enmeshed in clients' reciprocal webs of care and obligation. Through these relationships, care workers embody their clients' lifetimes of experience, thereby delivering the flexible care that sustains clients' independence. In the next chapter, I show how care workers' sensorially attuned bodily care draws on moral imagination learned among kin. Through this form of care, workers recognize older adults' subjectivity and generate their ongoing independence. In the process, bodily care intensifies social inequality.

4

Embodying Inequality

Empathy and Hierarchy in Daily Care

Sally Middleton and I sat one seat apart from each other in the windowless waiting area outside the emergency room of a small private hospital on Chicago's north side, our pile of heavy winter coats and overstuffed bags filling the seat in between. Though it was only early evening, the midwinter sun had set several hours earlier, making it feel much later. Or perhaps it was simply that we were weary and worried—it had already been a very long day and promised to grow longer still. The small ceiling-mounted television mumbled the evening news, casting blue light off the beige linoleum tiles and orange vinyl seats in the otherwise shadowy room. Sally fidgeted, her eyes darting eagerly each time someone passed, hoping it was a hospital staff person coming to tell us what was going on with Ms. Murphy, her client.

Around lunchtime earlier that day, Ms. Murphy had started coughing and gagging. Sally spent four hours a day, two days per week, helping Ms. Murphy with showers, laundry, cooking, and cleaning. That day—a Tuesday—Sally and I had been with Ms. Murphy for only about 30 minutes before she began coughing, which was enough time for Sally to lug the laundry down to the basement of the apartment building while Ms. Murphy told me what groceries she needed me to buy. By the time I returned from the store half an hour later, Ms. Murphy, still coughing, had started vomiting small amounts of viscous pink liquid. She could not catch her breath. With mounting panic in her eyes, Sally decided to call Ms. Murphy's doctor. The doctor's answering service told Sally to call 911, which sent an ambulance.

When Sally hung up the phone, Ms. Murphy told us that earlier in the morning she drank a glass of what she now thought might have been spoiled milk. Panting for air between each word, she said her stomach had soured a little while later. She had taken a dose (or maybe two) of cherry flavored Pepto-Bismol, explaining the candy-pink color of the liquid her body was expelling. Listening to Ms. Murphy recount the morning's events, a cloud came over Sally's face. As we rushed around the apartment preparing for the paramedic's arrival, Sally worried that she was inadvertently responsible for Ms. Murphy drinking spoiled milk.

Ms. Murphy had long since lost her sense of smell and was virtually unable to distinguish spoiling food from fresh using that sense alone. Ms. Murphy drank milk with every meal and as a snack several times throughout the day, reminded with each sip of her childhood on an Irish dairy farm. Ms. Murphy stockpiled pint size cartons of milk, regularly sending me to purchase more from the drugstore around the corner. She worried that she might run out of this source of sustenance, so essential to her sense of self, when no one was around to help her get more. Given the steady accumulation of open, partially empty milk cartons in the refrigerator, Sally made smelling and discarding any even slightly sour pints part of her regular routine.

Sally had been sick and missed work the week before Ms. Murphy fell ill, and thus it was possible that a carton of milk had spoiled in the meantime. After Ms. Murphy mentioned the possible cause of her distress, Sally went straight to the refrigerator, opening and sniffing cartons and discarding a half-empty one sitting at the front of the top shelf. There was no way to be sure, but Sally seemed convinced that it had been this carton that caused Ms. Murphy's upset stomach and the cascade of problems that followed.

Sally's habit of smelling Ms. Murphy's milk is one example of the hundreds of similarly quotidian acts of care home care workers perform that sustain the memories and personhood of clients like Ms. Murphy despite physical declines and social losses. These everyday care practices require workers to use their bodies to sensorially imagine and enact their clients' subjectivities, simultaneously generating elders' ways of life and subordinating their own well-being. By examining home care practices as simultaneously embodied, moral, and exploitative, this chapter considers the ways that bodily care generates both persons and hierarchies between them.

As a care worker, Sally did not seek to alter the rhythms of Ms. Murphy's daily life in either fundamental or mundane ways. Rather, she sought to sustain Ms. Murphy's life down to the smallest detail.

Sally could have sustained Ms. Murphy's health by substituting non-perishable nutrition drinks for milk. That Sally continued to purchase and then smell milk indicated she was trying to do more than simply sustain the older woman's life. To sustain Ms. Murphy's way of living, Sally cultivated an ability to use her own physical senses, emotions, and experiences to imagine the significance of Ms. Murphy's sensory history. She then drew on this embodied imagination to guide her home care practice. Drinking milk, made safe because Sally used her more capable body to stand in for Ms. Murphy's aging body, helped Ms. Murphy recognize herself. This embodied care enabled Ms. Murphy to feel that she was still the same person she had previously been, despite—or, rather, against—her diminished sense of smell and the ravaging pain of rheumatoid arthritis that had so limited her activity. It was Sally's deeply embodied labor that made it possible for Ms. Murphy to feel these continuities in her personhood.

At the heart of what both workers and older adults described as good care is workers' abilities to regenerate their clients' familiar ways of life. To accomplish this, home care workers engage their own bodies as the experiential ground for imagining and sustaining elders' lives.[1] As workers imagine the lived experiences, tastes, preferences, and routines of their clients, their imagination is not a purely mental exercise but also a sensorial one. Drawing on this form of imagining the lives of others, workers use their bodies as extensions of the older bodies of clients. In some cases, workers extend this embodied imaginative capacity still further, inhabiting the social roles and relationships absent from their elderly clients' lives. They hope to sustain elderly clients' ways of life and social personhoods along with their physical well-being.

Embodied practices in home care demand that workers quickly develop deep, intersubjective awareness of their clients' personalities, moods, and lifetimes of experience. They then combine these nuanced understandings of their clients with the pragmatic skills required to maintain elders' homes and daily routines. In the process, they transform seemingly straightforward tasks like cooking, cleaning, and grocery shopping into moral practices that help older adults feel like the persons they have always been. These practices generate older adults as independent persons who remain able to exert their will and shape the world around them according to their subjectivities.

Home care workers' everyday care sustains the personhoods of elderly clients by helping them live in a manner that both elders and those around them recognize as independent. In this context, independence is not a consequence of bounded bodies or self-determination. In practice, independence is a deeply relational form of personhood in which the generative labor and social hierarchies that sustain life are intentionally hidden and unreciprocal.[2]

Sally was about 15 years younger than her client. A thin woman whose pale skin was nearly translucent, Sally styled her gray hair in a halo of perfectly set curls framing her expressive blue eyes. She dressed simply and immaculately in perfectly ironed tan trousers and simple tops, wearing a floral smock to keep tidy while she worked. Sally had taken care of older adults for most of her adult life, first as the sole caregiver for her parents when her mother and then her father succumbed to chronic disease and debility. After her parents died, she moved to Chicago, to be closer to the Moody Bible church, whose radio programs had sustained her through the long years of her parents' illnesses. She soon became employed as a home care worker, living simply in one of the city's publicly subsidized senior apartment buildings. She did not drive, but rather used public transit and walked to and from her clients' homes in all weather. She loved her work, bringing to it the meticulous attention to detail and quiet efficiency she had honed over decades caring for kin. However, she found the physically demanding work of home care increasingly difficult. Though her Belltower supervisors were always trying to get her to take more clients, she cut back her hours, working only four hours a day, four days a week.[3] Still, she was sick more often than ever before, and sore nearly all the time. She worried that it was unfair to her clients to continue to care for them, fearing that she no longer had the bodily vigor necessary to sustain both her life and theirs.

Less than two weeks after Ms. Murphy returned from the hospital, Sally retired from home care work. Ms. Murphy took Sally's departure personally, feeling abandoned when she most needed support. Reconstructing what had happened after Ms. Murphy was released from the hospital through conversations with Belltower supervisors, Ms. Murphy, and Sally herself, I learned that Belltower had asked ("pressured" was the word Sally used) Sally to stay overnight at Ms. Murphy's apartment for the first several nights she was home from the hospital. The only place for Sally to sleep in the apartment was Ms. Murphy's long, nar-row sofa, which featured yellow upholstery and mid-century styling that suggested it had been in service since at least the late 1960s. Ms. Murphy was an agreeable patient, but she was weak and had to wake Sally up every time she used the bathroom. Between the interrupted sleep and the growing crick in her back from sleeping on the worn sofa, Sally told me she was barely able to walk after a few days. When the agency told her that Ms. Murphy was going to need eight hours of daily assistance even after overnight care ended, Sally prayed over her future, and de-cided that her time as a home care worker was over. Once Ms. Murphy was able to be on her own overnight, Sally abruptly informed her super-visors that she was retiring and her last day would be the following week.

The unraveling of Sally and Ms. Murphy's relationship highlights the deep and fragile entanglements between the lives and bodies of older adults and those of their home care workers. Focusing on everyday care practices, like Sally's vigilance over Ms. Murphy's milk cartons, shows how these practices involve a kind of embodied empathy that blurs the boundaries between older adults' and home care workers' bodies and their personhoods. At the same time, these practices generate some bod-ies and persons as taking priority over others. Sally's retirement shows that the priority placed on older adults' well-being contributes to the industry's broader instability by overlooking care workers' well-being. Through their care practices, care workers' bodies become the ground upon which moral hierarchies between persons—by which I mean the sense that some people's needs and desires ought to take priority over others'—were built, experienced, and justified on a day-to-day basis. Home care work leads to the embodiment of social hierarchies, shap-ing individual subjectivities and thereby making those hierarchies feel morally justified.[4]

In the process of sustaining older adults' ways of life, home care work-ers incorporate clients' histories of sensory experience into their own bodies while also working to limit their clients' exposure to their own ways of life. Home care workers' moral judgments and subjectivities come to reflect their repeated performance of acts that prioritize the bodily dispositions of elderly clients above their own. Home care work-ers see themselves as moral persons precisely because their embodied performances of social hierarchies enable them to sustain their older, often wealthier, clients' ways of life and independence. Thus, embodied care contributes to corporeal hierarchies in which poor women—and disproportionately women of color—are positioned to embody the felt values and sensory histories of their clients without the expectation that the moral worlds of their own sensorial landscapes will circulate in similar fashion.

Bodies at Care

Celia Tomas, Sally's supervisor at Belltower, told me about her experience working as a home care worker in Chicago right after she emigrated from the Philippines. Though she rarely spoke so directly to workers, the care ethics she shared with me permeated her supervisory interactions and were widely shared by care workers. Celia told me that putting clients' needs ahead of her own preferences was the only moral way to provide care. "I'm thinking I'm over here to work, I'm not thinking of my own comfort, I'm dancing to their [clients'] music. Maybe just because I came from another country, I wanted to impress them, but maybe also because from everyday life that's how you're supposed to do—you accepted the job and you really have to accept that you have to go down to the client's level." She continued, "When I came here I had to adapt and swallow my ego because it was a different environment, a different kind of job. If you're a good caregiver and doing a good job satisfying what they want is so easy, it's so easy to have them be satisfied, and then you develop rapport. So it's important to accept your job and accept your client when they are scolding you, it's not because you're a low-class worker, but because they are sick." Celia's metaphor of "dancing to their music" deftly communicates an understanding of care as a form of bodily attention and accommodation to the needs of another. Celia understood her participation in the bodily hierarchies created by care as a fundamentally moral act, what "you're supposed to do." Though Celia recognized the role that social inequality played in placing poor women, and immigrant women, in these jobs, she argued that their subservient role was morally justified by older adults' physical vulnerability. Like Celia, home care workers saw themselves as moral persons precisely because they were able to put their clients' needs above their own, sustaining elders' sense of independence while bearing the bodily and social costs of both these intimate hierarchies and broader social inequalities.

Understanding the ways that care labor generates embodied persons and hierarchies requires rethinking common Euro-American understandings of bodies. For centuries, common-sense Euro-American notions of the body have reflected Platonic and Enlightenment philosophies that view the material world as fundamentally separate from the social, psychological, spiritual, and moral aspects of life. These Cartesian dualities profoundly impact understandings of the body as distinct from the mind, for example, or the natural world as separate from the social world. Social theorist Pierre Bourdieu argues that Enlightenment philosophies often pose the body, with its messy emotions and senses, as opposed to rational thought and as a "hindrance to knowledge."[5] Enlightenment philosophies also posit the body as the unit of the individual, independent person. Anthropologists Judith Farquhar and Margaret Lock describe this as the idea of the "body proper" which "has been treated as a skin bound, rights bearing, communicating, experiencing, biomechanical entity."[6] As such, societies influenced by the Enlightenment came to understand the body proper as the container of personhood and the unit of citizenship. This way of thinking posits the body as the material foundation of social life, delimiting the possibilities for both individuals and societies.

Contrary to Cartesian philosophy, social and physical scientists have shown that human bodies are not simply raw material upon which social life depends. Rather, human bodily development requires human social worlds to proceed, and human relationships and environments profoundly influence what kinds of bodies develop. Actions as simple and common as sitting, bathing, and toileting vary significantly around the world—evidence that the body techniques for each of these activities are transmitted through social means rather than being direct products of physiology.[7] Though humans have a biological capacity for language, babies and young children excluded from human communities never develop the ability to use language. Similarly, social emphasis on particular kinds of bodily senses and skills strengthens those capacities, transmitting moral values by bodily means.[8] For example, in the United States (unlike much of the world), parents often expect babies and young children to sleep alone. Solitary sleep is thought to teach babies the bodily and emotional regulation necessary for independent personhood.[9] As these cases show, human bodies are inseparable from the relations and environments they shape and are shaped by.

From this point of view, bodies are simultaneously social and natural, discursive and material, subject and object.[10] Understood this way, bodies are not simply containers for human rationalities but rather a mutable, contingent medium that simultaneously reflects and generates social and historical contexts. Social scientists use the term "embodiment" to describe the processual making and doing of bodies, instead of conceiving of bodies as a pre-social object for analysis.[11] As suggested in the example of American infant sleep practices, persons are constantly being generated through repeated bodily practices. Through these kinds of bodily habits, individual people come to share embodied dispositions with others around them—they tend to like similar kinds of food, music, etc., share similar forms of posture, ways of dressing, and even show similar skill at activities like dancing or carrying objects on their heads. Social scientists use the term "habitus" to describe the corpus of these embodied/moral dispositions. Bourdieu argues that habitus is both generated by and generative of everyday behavior and broader social structures.[12] Because habitus is inculcated through everyday practice, communities that collaborate in making daily life possible generally share habitus.[13] As such, people from similar geographic, class, ethnic, generational, religious, etc., backgrounds tend to share dispositions, finding similar things pleasurable or disgusting, polite or rude, right or wrong.

The notions of embodied practice and habitus are useful for analyzing how processes of embodiment are implicated in social inequality. The habitus prominent in powerful communities tend to become socially dominant, while those of disadvantaged groups are cast as inferior. Often, the failure of those from non-dominant groups to embody the habitus of more powerful groups is used to justify their disadvantage and exclude them from opportunity.[14] Recall from chapter 3, for example, how supervisor Carmen Rodriguez judged Daronda's sartorial choices, faulting a job applicant for not having developed middle-class sensibilities regarding professional attire.

Embodiment is ongoing across the life course, as people engage in intertwined biological, environmental, and social processes. Human bodies are continually generated by human labor, especially through the kinds of practices Americans refer to as "care."[15] While discussions of embodiment often focus on earlier life, people continue to develop ways of being in and experiencing the world as they grow older. For example, many older adults experience diminished senses—not only vision and hearing but also taste and smell. These changes can radically alter their embodied experience of daily life. Many older adults in Chicago responded to sensory changes by focusing on their histories of experience with specific activities. Thus, many older adults continued to find pleasure in things they had previously enjoyed, regardless of whether their sensorial engagements with those things remained constant. For example, Mrs. Silverman told me that she continued to eat familiar foods, despite not being able to taste them or even remember how they tasted, because "even though I can't really taste anything, if I didn't like it before, I don't like it now. I know it's silly, but I still don't like the things I didn't like. I won't even try them. I've always been kind of a picky eater, so I still am." Being a picky eater was important to Mrs. Silverman's subjectivity, so she continued to eat the foods she had enjoyed earlier in life.

Home care workers recognize the importance of this kind of bodily continuity to older adults. They strive to provide continuity in their elderly clients' histories of experience, generating daily routines through their care practices that reflect their clients' habitus. For example, Grace Washington sometimes substituted as a live-in care worker for a woman named Lillian, who was dying. Lillian was Polish, and on the weekend, her ten children visited, bringing a feast of "pierogi and stuffed cabbage and sausage with sauerkraut and some kind of meat that looked like sliced roast beef, and potato pancakes." Grace had not eaten Polish food before, but told me it was "really good, especially those pierogi and potato pancakes." Lillian was losing her ability to chew and swallow, so all her food had to be mashed or blended. Lillian's children offered to purchase baby food so it would be easier for care workers to feed her, but Grace would not hear of it. "Lillian loves to eat, so we can't feed her baby food. She's not a baby! Instead, I just blend up her regular food and I leave it a little bit thick so that she can still feel the texture and taste those things. When the family came over they brought all the Polish food Lillian likes and were visiting. She didn't eat much of the soup they were trying to feed her, but when I blended up those pierogis, she ate those up just fine." In taking the extra time to blend foods with which Lillian was familiar, Grace recognized that providing older adults with sustenance meant more than providing calories. It also meant recognizing that her clients were not babies with unformed palates but older people with lifetimes of experience that shaped their tastes and habits. By attuning care to the sensory aspects of habitus, for example taste and smell, home care workers are able provide older adults with sustenance, with experiences that sustain their personhood along with their bodies.

Maria Arellano told me that this attunement to clients' different embodied histories was at the heart of good care. "That is one of the things I certainly love about working with the elderly. Your true self comes at a certain age. I feel that if you live so long, every body is a person of their own." She explained her statement by telling me how she cared for memorable clients, "I had a gentleman, his name was Milton. He never married 'cause he made a success of just taking care of his family. His mom you know after his father died. His brothers, his sister you know, and his sisters took care of him by hiring me . . . I used to take him for long walks. I would always try to find that little thing that person likes. And him being in the navy would be the water. So I would drive him to the beach so he could watch the kids. Went to the lake and just watched the boats. He liked to take baths, so I would make sure his showers were a little longer."

"And then I had this other lady, she must have been some lady when she was young. She was always telling me about her sex life and dating and oh my God. She would turn you red. She was wonderful . . . They pretty much tell you what their thing is if you give them half a chance. Because they tell you what their surroundings was. Was it religious? Was it parties? Was it a home life? . . . Okay whatever it was, you find that. Okay. With Mr. M it was the beach. With Mrs. C it was food. She loved food so I found her special dinners. With Ms. J it was company. Men. So I would make sure when I came to visit once in awhile, I would bring one of my boys and that would just bring a smile to her face. You know. Or I would invite a neighbor over for tea for her. Course with my company and that always brought a smile . . . With Ms. Silverman, I could just. . . . I took her out for a walk and it makes her shine."

Maria listened to her clients talk about their lives, searching for key experiences that made each client feel like "a person of their own." Each of the examples she gave focused on the sensorial and social aspects of her clients' embodied histories—taking long baths, watching boats, flirting with men. To make clients shine required more than cooking and cleaning, it meant attuning care to the sensorial aspects of a client's life. It meant helping clients feel, in their bodies, continuity between their earlier life and current experience.

Despite residing in the same city, older adults and workers were likely to have different embodied dispositions, as their habitus were shaped by their different backgrounds and generational histories. Even workers and older adults who might on the surface appear to be from similar communities only partially shared habitus. For example, black American workers and older adults, both living in Chicago's South Side, might both wipe down their bathroom sinks before exiting the washroom but disagree about the proper way to cook classic Southern dishes due to different migration and familial histories. To sustain older adults' ways of life, home care workers learn to embody their clients' dispositions, coming to sense when bathwater is the right temperature, when a dish is adequately salty or sweet, and when a social outing will lift their client's mood. On a daily basis, home care requires workers to use their bodies to imagine the embodied experiences of their elderly clients, and then prioritize older adults' bodily dispositions above their own. Through this daily practice of subsuming their bodily comfort in order to care for others, home care workers come to feel, quite literally, the broader hierarchies structuring home care work.

Embodying Moral Relations

Kim Little always entered George Sampson's apartment with a flurry of activity, flinging herself through the door. With her bustle and cheerful hello, Kim broke the calm that otherwise filled the apartment. Often, I would arrive a few minutes before Kim, sitting quietly while Mr. Sampson finished a phone conversation. The Moody Bible radio station was nearly always on, playing softly in the background. During his married life, Mr. Sampson had been a religious man, but working two and three jobs at a time as a waiter and hospital custodian had left him little time for bible study. One of the blessings of retirement had been attending Moody's bible study groups. Now that he was too frail to go out, he continued to learn and worship via their radio programs.

The multiple tote bags and purses Kim carried overwhelmed her slight frame, filling the small entryway as she tumbled inside. By the time she arrived at Mr. Sampson's apartment early each afternoon, she had already traveled dozens of miles back and forth across the city on public buses, first dropping her children off at school before heading to her appointments with other home care clients. She carried supplies for these journeys with her—lunch, a change of clothes, several water bottles, deodorant, toiletries, a book and so on. At least once a week, she stopped in the middle of her bus ride to Mr. Sampson's home to buy him the brand of frozen fish he liked from the discount grocery that carried it for several dollars less than his neighborhood store. Mr. Sampson could not really afford to eat fish at full price, and it was one of the few dishes he enjoyed that also met his doctor's recommendations for diabetic-friendly, low-sodium meals. Kim insisted the extra stop was no trouble, but even when the buses ran on time (a rarity), it added a good 20 minutes to her already long days. Mr. Sampson lived in a publicly subsidized senior housing building only a few blocks from Chicago's magnificent mile, and the grocery stores nearby were aimed at the neighborhood's more affluent population. The building's many black American residents and care providers, including Mr. Sampson and Kim, stood out in the predominately white neighborhood.

Through her job with Plusmore, Kim had grown used to working with clients with limited budgets. She knew how much difference buying at discount could make for both their finances and their health. Sometimes on her way home, she stopped again at the discount grocery to buy food for her family. She shared a house with several siblings and her children. Their shared economic situation was also deeply precarious. This did not stop Kim from dreaming of a better economic future. One afternoon after work, she took me to see the handbag she had fallen in love with at one of the luxury stores a few blocks from Mr. Sampson's apartment. Unfazed by the price tag in the thousands of dollars, Kim swore one day she would find a way to own one.

As soon as Kim set down her bags and put the groceries away, she and Mr. Sampson began their daily tête-à-tête to figure out what she could make him for lunch and dinner that he would actually eat. Each day, Kim opened with the same question: "You hungry?" His answer a foregone conclusion: "Yeah, but I don't have the taste for anything."

Facing each other in the small apartment entryway, she closed her eyes and smacked her lips as she thought out loud: "yesterday you had fried chicken, maybe you want meatballs today?" He dithered, unable to decide, as nothing ever sounded appetizing the first time through. Kim continued to offer suggestions. She could almost always sense what he wanted to eat based on the rhythms of his appetite and the ways it shifted in relation to his energy, mood, and the weather. Often, however, he rejected her first suggestion out-of-hand, so she'd offer a few more choices and then circle back to the first.

Kim usually stopped at two or three neighborhood stores on her nearly daily grocery runs for Mr. Sampson. If Mr. Sampson decided on meatballs for lunch, she quickly ran to the Italian restaurant that made them the way he liked and placed an order, promising to return in half an hour to pick them up. Then she would head over to the grocery store to pick up the majority of items that Mr. Sampson liked, getting each item on the list. For some groceries, she could get whichever brand was on sale, but for some food Mr. Sampson only liked one brand. So, she lugged the groceries several blocks to the convenience store. There, she purchased the specific brand and flavor of fried pork skins and brand of diet lemon-lime soda that Mr. Sampson liked. The grocery didn't carry the first item, and the second was substantially less expensive at the convenience store. Now carrying another heavy bag, Kim rushed another block back to the restaurant to pick up Mr. Sampson's lunch. She hurried back to his apartment so she could prepare his meal before it got cold.

During one of these trips, Kim admitted that she had started planning the heavier runs around my visits, saving the purchase of bottled drinks and heavy glass jars for when she had someone to help her carry them. For a while, she paid some of the homeless men who hung out around the nearby El train stop a dollar or two to help her get her groceries back to the building. When Mr. Sampson found out, he yelled at her for talking with strange men. He could be so overprotective, she told me.

Even though Kim disagreed with Mr. Sampson, she had stopped interacting with the homeless men. In acceding to his wishes, she deployed forms of moral imagination which recognized Mr. Sampson as a particular kind of person—male, authoritarian, protective—and comported herself in ways that enabled him to continue to experience himself this way. Though she would have preferred not to carry the heavy bags by herself, she adjusted—making multiple small runs, waiting for me to show up, and when all else failed, hauling the heavy groceries herself. In this sense, when pushed, Kim chose to provide care that strengthened Mr. Sampson's subjectivity over her bodily well-being.

After she put the groceries away, Kim reheated the lunch she had purchased during her errands, often supplementing it with a side dish she knew he'd like—a frozen waffle or cornbread. At the same time, she started preparing Mr. Sampson's supper, chopping greens, mixing batter, or defrosting fish. Cooking for Mr. Sampson was a challenge. His diabetes and other ailments created numerous food restrictions, which made most recipes bland and unpalatable. Mr. Sampson compared Kim's cooking to his mother's. He said, "I'm used to good cooking, but it's [Kim's cooking] eatable. Especially when I'm ill like I've been, that's the only food you are going to get." Nothing, not even his wife's cooking, had really been up to his standards, which he said were set by his mother, who "could cook everything. She was a terrific cook, and I liked everything she made. I remember at home we had this big glass front cabinet and it would always be full of pies and cakes and cookies and donuts. She could cook anything. All the guys at school would want to come over to my house to eat." Kim could not compete. Nevertheless, as she cooked, Kim diligently tested the food, incorporating his feedback on her previous attempts and trying to imagine the tastes and textures from Mr. Sampson's childhood memories. Though her cooking never measured up to those memories, her efforts at least rendered the food edible.

Notably, Mr. Sampson imagined Kim as filling multiple female kin roles. Sometimes he protected her like he might a daughter or wife, but sometimes he saw her as filling a maternal role. Kim, he told me, did not live up to his own mother's standards, but he still preferred her to anyone else. On the rare days when Kim had to miss work because one of her children was sick or had a doctor's appointment, Mr. Sampson almost always declined the agency's offer of a substitute worker. It just was not worth it for him to have someone in the house that did not know what he liked to eat or where things went.

Once Mr. Sampson's lunch was ready, Kim placed a small folding table at the edge of Mr. Sampson's bed, setting it neatly with a folded napkin, silverware, a glass of water, and a glass of diet 7-Up. As Mr. Sampson ate, Kim sat on a small stool in the corner of his bedroom. She propped her back against the windowsill, hastily drinking the large bottle of water and nibbling at the lunch she brought from home. Before they started eating, Mr. Sampson led them in a short prayer, asking for God's blessings over the food, ending with a quick refrain, "only God is good ALL the time," which Kim echoed, "ALL the time."

After praying, they watched courtroom television shows. *Judge Mathis*, an African American Chicagoan, was their favorite, but *Family Court* was good too. As they watched together, they discussed the cases and sometimes shouted loudly at the litigants in the courtroom. For example, one afternoon, the case involved a disagreement between two friends over a $3,000 loan. As the judge patiently questioned the plaintiff, Mr. Sampson guffawed, saying he would never loan anyone $3,000, and if he did, he would certainly have to make sure to get the loan documented on paper. Kim agreed, saying that "it would have to be signed and sealed and notarized or I'd never lend that much money." Mr. Sampson laughed, saying that "you loan money to a friend, but you get it back from an enemy." Kim nodded, laughing in agreement. Mr. Sampson disparaged the plaintiff's pinstripe suit, striped shirt, and striped tie as mismatched and too busy, which he took to be a sign that the man was superficial and had bad taste: "more money than sense." Kim asked Mr. Sampson if he thought the defendant who had borrowed the money was "playing senile. Like how would he not know if he had paid the loan back, after 30 years, you gotta know if you paid or not." As they ate, watched, and talked, Mr. Sampson's face lit up and became animated, a stark contrast to his normally reserved demeanor.

After the physically exhausting commute and grocery shopping, Kim relished the opportunity to get off of her feet for a few minutes. Yet this was no break. As they sat and talked with the television, Kim and Mr. Sampson forged a moral community, debating the norms of correct behavior and means of enforcing them. By praying and watching judge shows with Mr. Sampson, Kim inhabited a daughterly role, enabling Mr. Sampson to continue to inhabit a fatherly one. Together, they created a social world in which Mr. Sampson could share his religious and paternal concern over right action. No longer able to attend church or teach Sunday school, Mr. Sampson had limited engagement with these kinds of communities. His lunches with Kim became one of the few moments in which to enact this aspect of his social personhood. Though Kim could not fully reproduce the culinary and housekeeping skill of Mr. Sampson's mother, she supported him as a protective, authoritarian, and paternal person by comporting herself in a daughterly manner, receiving his moral and practical instruction about how to behave both within and beyond the household.

Kim was exquisitely attuned to Mr. Sampson's bodily rhythms and habits. Her attention was itself a body technique—a learned way of using her body to imagine how Mr. Sampson was feeling and then act in ways that would bring him comfort. This form of care not only required Kim to learn new ways to cook and keep house, but also to accommodate Mr. Sampson's paternal concerns even though doing so made her job even more physically taxing. Through her generative labor, Kim enabled Mr. Sampson to continue to live as the moral, masculine person he understood himself to be. By sustaining these aspects of Mr. Sampson's subjectivity, Kim sustained Mr. Sampson's independence.

Embodying Social Lives

Home care workers draw on embodied imagination to sustain clients' social relations. In many contexts, shared meals have the power to constitute both persons and their relations. For the older adults I knew in Chicago, meals often threatened to become visceral, routine moments of loss, nostalgia, and loneliness, in part because of the sensory reminders infusing food and the relentless need to eat. Home care workers do what they can to mitigate these losses, offering themselves as fleshy, imperfect specters of the fathers, mothers, wives, husbands, children, and friends who have previously prepared and eaten meals with clients. Workers consciously comport their bodies in ways that reflect older adults' previous relations through the clothes they wear, the food they eat, and the kinds of conversations in which they engage. In so doing, home care workers sustain both the social and sensorial tenor of older adults' lives.

John Thomas, a 95-year-old Belltower client of German descent, told me that before Doris Robinson came to work with him several years earlier, he had lost a worrisome amount of weight. Mr. Thomas resisted hiring a home care worker for two years after his wife died, despite regular pleas from his son, his neighbor, and a social worker at the nearby senior center. He had always been strong, making a living off his fitness and his double black belt in judo. When he first came to Chicago, he lived at the YMCA. There, he met a Japanese man with whom he traded swimming lessons for judo lessons. He found it a strange twist of history that a few years later he used his judo training to teach hand-to-hand combat to train navy sailors bound for the war against Japan. At age 95, he still rode his stationary bike five miles each morning—a concession to safety made after he fell during one of his daily 20-mile rides outdoors several years earlier. Then he fell again carrying the laundry downstairs. Ever focused on his health, the falls and the weight loss had finally convinced Mr. Thomas to hire a home care worker.

Mr. Thomas had been married for 65 years. After his wife passed away, he lost interest in cooking and eating. Cooking had become a painful reminder of their early years together, when he taught his bride to cook. Raised in Tennessee, Mrs. Thomas's family had black domestic workers, and she had not been prepared to fill the role of a northern middle-class housewife. Mr. Thomas, raised by a widowed mother who was a custodian for a state prison in Pennsylvania (and lived on the grounds), had learned to cook and clean as a young boy. Once his wife had gotten the hang of cooking, he rarely did so again. For most of his adult life, Mr. Thomas focused on his career as a debt collector for one of Chicago's large candy companies. Mr. Thomas resumed cooking only in the last years of his wife's life, preparing all of her favorite dishes, until eventually she could only eat grits and soup. After she died, he simply could not face returning to the kitchen.

Instead, Mr. Thomas began eating breakfast at Seven Brothers, a family restaurant where he and his wife had gone for Sunday brunch after attending church for decades. When Doris came to work with him, he included her in this routine, eventually extending the invitation to me. He drove the three of us the six miles from his home to the restaurant in his 1980s Oldsmobile. He insisted on driving, since he was sure that, "if I stop, they'll never let me start again, and then what would I do?" Besides, he was still a safer driver than most people he knew. Recognizing that these meals were the highlight of his day, Doris arrived for work each morning dressed for the occasion. She wore a skirt, blouse, and high-heeled shoes, imitating the formality of those earlier breakfasts shared with his wife. He ordered nearly the same thing each day: scrambled eggs, toast, bacon, and fruit.

During the meal, Mr. Thomas sat quietly, a gentle, bemused smile on his face as he listened to Doris's stories about her daughters, grandchildren, distant relatives, and neighbors. I learned later from Mr. Thomas's son that Mrs. Thomas had been something of a gossip, always ready with a juicy story to tell. Mr. Thomas told me one of the things he most appreciated about Doris was that she always had interesting things to share, and he seemed to take great pleasure in being able to listen to a woman dissect her social world once more. With her chattering away, he finished his plate each morning. Through these deeply gendered conversations, Doris and Mr. Thomas created a moral community reminiscent of those Mr. Thomas had been part of earlier in life.

When we returned from breakfast, Doris changed into scrubs and gym shoes—attire more appropriate for cleaning and cooking. Doris never sought to replace Mr. Thomas's wife, but her body techniques allowed her to occupy a wifely role. With Doris at his side, Mr. Thomas could continue to play the familiar role of the patient, attentive audience to a socially engaged, chatty woman. Through her dress and gossip, Doris embodied and sustained the social and material tenor of Mr. Thomas's prior relationship. Though the subject matter and tenor differed significantly from Kim Little and George Sampson's commentary about TV courtroom dramas, both pairs created moral communities reminiscent of the client's earlier social worlds through daily mealtime conversations.

Mrs. Silverman had been widowed for nearly 30 years by the time we met and no longer yearned for meals with her husband. Instead, she grieved the loss of her regular lunches with friends and neighbors— many of whom had died or whose mobility was as limited as her own. Being able to get out of the house to run errands and eat lunch at McDonald's was the highlight of her visits with her home care worker Maria Arellano (and me). Maria had the routine for lunch at McDonald's down pat—she would help Mrs. Silverman find a quiet seat away from any noisy children, so that the older woman would be able to participate in conversation even if she had "forgotten" to wear her despised hearing aids (perhaps intentionally, as she, like many older adults, hated them).

Once Mrs. Silverman was seated, Maria and I went to the counter to order our meals. Maria assiduously avoided fatty and fried foods and never ate at fast-food restaurants in her non-work life. She joked with me that she always ordered a filet-o-fish because she had researched the

McDonald's menu and decided it was "the least unhealthy" item on the menu, though "none of them are actually healthy." Despite her objections, Maria ate at McDonald's with Mrs. Silverman regularly because she understood how important these shared meals were to Mrs. Silverman. She did her best to accommodate her client's desires while protecting her own health by always ordering the fish sandwich because this was just another aspect of making her client "shine." One of the prerogatives of old age, she told me, was getting to do what you wanted. "If you live so long, you deserve to do so much. Nobody should be able to tell you what to do." Of course, this meant that Maria temporarily surrendered control over what she ate to please her clients. Good care, Maria told me, required one to place more emphasis on "what they need and not how you feel."

As home care workers eat alongside their clients, they embody the social roles that make their elderly clients feel like themselves. In so doing, home care workers adopt bodily habits different from their own. They eat food they might otherwise avoid, wear clothing in which they would not otherwise work, and debate television shows they might otherwise ignore. Inhabiting the embodied dispositions of dead spouses, unavailable friends, distant kin, workers set aside their own comfort and dispositions to sustain their clients' social personhood.

Naturalizing Inequality

Workers also articulate a sense of their own moral value as stemming from their willingness and ability to prioritize others' bodily needs and social desires above their own. In so doing, they endorse the virtues espoused in home care worker training programs that "the client's needs come first." Workers recognize that providing this form of "good care" might require them to experience bodily discomfort, disgust, or even danger. Even as they embody their clients' ways of life, they accept that their own sensorial preferences and social backgrounds should not circulate into older adults' homes. In this way, everyday home care practices generate embodied hierarchies in which it feels morally appropriate that older people's preferences and desires take priority over those of their care workers.

Care workers frequently rely on idioms of the body to describe their ability to prioritize their clients' social and sensory worlds over their own feelings. They describe these bodily accommodations as being at the heart of good care. Grace Washington told me that even though it could be frustrating to listen to clients tell the same stories over and over "When you are in this kind of life, they get like that, and you just learn to bend a little, take a little and adjust." When Mr. Sampson insulted Kim or acted in a manner she found condescending, she focused on empathically imagining his point of view rather than becoming angry. "I try to control myself and say [to myself] what is going on? What is he thinking about? I have to catch myself." Using the language of bodily manipulation—"dance to their tune," "bend a little," "catch myself"—workers emphasize the embodied nature of the empathic practices that enable them to sustain elders' ways of life even when these come into conflict with their own.

Care workers accept that they frequently work in homes that are uncomfortable and sometimes unhealthy because of their commitment to sustaining clients' physical health and personhood. For example, they repeatedly told me about their frustrations trying to clean and cook in apartments that elders routinely kept warm and unventilated, even on hot summer days. Aware that lowering the temperature or opening a window might make their clients uncomfortably chilly or even lead to illness, workers managed their own discomfort as best they could. In the winter, workers wore many layers to clients' homes, shedding layers of outerwear and sweaters to work in lightweight short sleeve shirts. Nearly every care worker I knew carried several bottles of water or soda with her to work, another means of trying to protect their health while doing heavy physical work in warm homes.

On occasion, the sensorial discomforts and bodily risks posed by an elder's home were more severe. Grace Washington's efforts to care for Margee Jefferson in one such circumstance exemplified the embodied empathy and dedication workers and older adults alike associated with good care. Margee's children hired Belltower to care for their mother after Margee tripped and fell. Unable to get up, she lay on the floor for several hours before her son came home and helped her up. The home itself had been the most significant challenge to her well-being. Belltower supervisors described Margee as a "severe hoarder" and noted that hers were by far the worst living conditions they had encountered. Grace worked tirelessly in these challenging conditions, striving to make the home safe but still familiar to her client.

Margee's home was filled to the brim with the collected belongings of three generations of continuous habitation. Margee's husband had been raised in the house, a stately two-story brick home in a serene neighborhood. After getting married, they lived for a few years in a small apartment. After their eldest son was born, they moved back into the home on the far west side of Chicago, sharing it with Margee's in-laws until the elder couple passed away. It was not clear which of the inhabitants had been responsible for the immense accumulation of belongings.

Grace and her supervisor, Carmen, had an ongoing disagreement about the best way to care for Margee. Carmen instructed Grace to impose a strict routine on Margee's day. Margee typically woke up early in the morning so her son could give her an insulin shot before he left for work. Then Margee went back to sleep, waking around eleven in the morning. Margee spent most of the day wearing a nightgown and robe. She changed into street clothes toward the evening in hopes that her son would take her to a restaurant for supper. Neither of them were very good cooks, and they either ate microwaveable meals or dined out every night. Carmen wanted Grace to awaken Margee by eight o'clock each morning, sponge bathe her and dress her in proper clothing before breakfast. Carmen instructed Grace to soak Margee's feet for at least half an hour each day. She also insisted that Grace alter Margee's diet by limiting the amount of cereal, bananas, and sugar Margee consumed. Instead, she instructed Grace to serve Margee warm lunches, soups, and diet microwave meals.

Grace disagreed with Carmen's instructions. She told me, "They're old. You can't come in here and say, 'Baby, you got to get up at 7:00 a.m.' . . . I let them keep with their daily routine. It may be modified a bit, but I'm not trying to modify it too much where it gets kind of confusing." To find the balance between subtle modification and confusing changes, Grace empathically imagined what it was like to be Margee's embodied self, reaching across differences of age, race, class, and lifetimes of experience to understand what alterations could be made without disrupting Margee's way of life. The work of sustaining Margee's independence and way of life required Grace to inhabit her own body differently. Grace used this imaginative, embodied attunement to make minor changes to Margee's home and meals, all the while challenging her supervisor's instructions to completely alter Margee's way of life.

In practice, this meant surreptitiously replacing the sugar in Margee's sugar bowl with a no-calorie sugar substitute, but continuing to provide the older woman with her preferred bananas and cereal. Grace explained to me that she could change the sugar without upsetting Margee because the taste and texture of the substitute were so similar, but there was no breakfast other than bananas and cereal that would satisfy the older woman. Similarly, Grace created some daily routines, encouraging Margee to rise and sit at the sunny dining room table around lunchtime by enthusiastically listening to Margee's oft-repeated stories. However, she refused to force Margee to wake up at eight in the morning and get dressed. Grace argued that if Margee wanted to sleep until eleven, that was her business. As Grace told me, "I have a problem with some of the company's rules." She continued, "So I'm supposed to go in there and tell her, 'Well, you got to get up because the boss says you got to get up.' Mind you, this is that lady's house. I'm a strong believer of . . . I'm younger than her. How am I going to come in here into your house and tell you when and where you got to put your clothes on?"

Grace argued, "As long as I have you up and dressed before my shift is over and have everything done, I don't see where there's a problem. . . . They got medical problems as is, so you've got to work with both hands." In these statements, Grace suggested that the ethical value of care was found in managing the tension between the competing moral goods, for example between implementing the medically prescribed dietary regimens and protecting the familiar routines that enable older adults to recognize their own lives.[16] Grace's insistence on protecting Margee's ability to control what happened in her home reflected widespread American ideologies about the relationship between private property and personhood. By embodying Margee's very different way of life, Grace subordinated her body to Margee's frailer body, enabling Margee to remain at home, and sustained her sense of independence.

As Grace Washington worked to sustain Margee Jefferson's routine and independence, she did so in Margee's sensorially overwhelming home. As Grace told me, when she first started working there, "the goddamn house wasn't fit for a dog to live in. . . . You got a room literally with garbage damn near filled to the ceiling. . . . Baby, if a dog went in that bathroom, the dog would turn around and walk away. . . . You got mold coming out the sink, whereas it looks like spiders is in infestation." Despite the hundreds of hours Grace and other Belltower workers had since spent clearing the home of debris, it remained a difficult place to work. The downstairs bathroom, which they had cleaned for hours, still did not meet Grace's standards of cleanliness. Grace used the toilet as little as possible when she was there, despite working 10-hour days with 2-hour commutes on each end. She told me, "I'm usually dancing at the door by the time I get home, I have to go so bad. But I'm drinking soda all day when I'm at Margee's home, so by the time I get to my house I'm running in the door. Some days it's so bad I call my husband when I get off the bus and ask him to open the door so I can come running in. If I really have to go at Margee's, I spray down the toilet several times with bleach, but it smells so bad in there no matter what I do." Nevertheless, she told me, "I didn't complain and I didn't have a problem with that because when I go into a senior's house, I take it as if this is my grandmother."

Grace's comparison between caring for clients and caring for kin was apt. Much as Grace accepted that her father continued to drink despite his poor health, she accepted the state of Margee's home. She did not particularly like either older adult's lifestyle, but she saw her role as their junior and as their carer to help them feel like independent persons who were still in control of their routines and homes. Grace was concerned about the effects on her health of spending so much time at Margee's home. Yet she believed it was her moral obligation as a care worker to stay and do what she could to protect her client's way of life and improve her well-being.

Care workers labor among and consume their clients' sensorial worlds. Sustaining their clients' ways of life and independence also means that carers work to prevent the intrusion of their own sensorial worlds into those of their clients. Agencies exhort workers to bathe every day, never wear unwashed clothes, and carry deodorant so clients will not have to smell body odors that might develop. Live-in workers are advised not to cook or bring "ethnic" food that might leave strange odors in clients' homes. For care workers, caring means subjecting their bodies to their clients' sensory worlds while limiting clients' exposure to their own worlds and lives.

For example, as Thanksgiving approached, Grace worried that the restaurant that Margee and her son favored would be closed for the holiday. Wanting to make sure Margee would still be able to celebrate in traditional fashion, Grace brought Margee several plates of the special Thanksgiving delicacies she had cooked in preparation for her own family's feast. The dishes were Southern-style recipes she had learned to cook from her mother rather than the German-style cooking Margee was accustomed to. Nevertheless, they included many foods she knew Margee liked. Grace cooked for weeks preparing for the holiday, an expression of the love and care she felt for her family and extended to Margee. There was so much food—candied sweet potatoes, barbeque ribs, smoked turkey, macaroni and cheese, cornbread, pecan pie, and pumpkin pie. When I next visited the pair a week after the Thanksgiving, the plates that Grace brought sat in the refrigerator untouched. Margee suggested that I should eat them, since no one else was going to. Grace looked down, disappointed but not surprised, and shrugged. Someone should enjoy the food, she said. As Margee ate her standard cereal-and-banana lunch, I could only finish a small portion of the still-delicious meal. While Grace spent 11 hours a day in Margee's overwhelming home, attuning her body to Margee's embodied tastes and daily rhythms, neither she nor Margee felt that the older woman was morally obliged to similarly partake in Grace's life. Rather than take for granted that this kind of bodily asymmetry is a natural part of relationships between care workers and those for whom they care, it is important to attend to the ways that these asymmetries are connected to ideologies of independence. Everyday care practices have profound moral stakes for both older adults and care workers because of their potential to either generate or corrode personhood. To sustain elders' lives in ways that reflect their bodily dispositions, care workers develop embodied knowledge of their clients' histories of experience. They then use their bodies to stand in for elders' bodies or to mimic elders' past relationships. In this way, workers' bodies serve as extensions of elders' bodies, mediating social and material interactions so that elders can continue to live in material worlds that reflect their subjectivities. Through these processes, independent personhood is constituted through bodily relations dependent on intimate and deeply hierarchical embodied relations.

While home care practices sustain elders' personhood, they also position care workers as persons whose social value lies in their willingness to suppress their subjective preferences in deference to those they care for. Viewed within the limited domain of the care interaction, the hierarchies of sensory knowledge generated in care practices appear legitimate, particularly since they play a significant role in maintaining elders' well-being and personhood. Yet viewed within the broader structures that shape home care work, these intimate hierarchies exacerbate social inequality. While workers come to intimately experience their clients' socially inculcated dispositions, the circulation of their own embodied ways of life is intentionally limited. Those who control workers' labor, including older adults, agency personnel, and policy makers, are not similarly positioned to develop empathic knowledge of the embodied toll exacted by home care labor and magnified by the instability produced by low wages and lack of benefits. The bodily hierarchies that appear moral in paid home care depend on, but also generate, a social world in which the lives of vulnerable older adults matter more than the lives of poor women of color.

Even as workers sustain older adults' independence, they are publicly constructed as "dependent" and thus as lesser persons by virtue of their need to supplement paltry wages and nonexistent benefits with government assistance. Home care agencies invest little in workers' bodily well-being, despite the centrality of workers' bodies to care. Without health insurance, workers regularly delay seeking medical care when they are ill—sometimes with significant consequences (for example, Doris delaying treatment for lupus). Without the benefit of paid sick leave, workers who are ill face an impossible choice between missing work and being unable to pay their bills or going to work and potentially passing an infection to a frail client. Positioned in such a way that they sometimes feel they cannot both prioritize their own needs and provide care in a moral manner, these workers frequently choose to act as moral persons and caring individuals.[17] However, the bodily toll of this form of care accumulates. Workers who can find other means of supporting themselves and their kin, like Sally, eventually quit.

Home care workers maintain older adults' homes as one critical extension of the ways that they use their bodies to sustain clients' subjectivities. The next chapter shows how home care workers materially produce the conditions of older adults' independence through everyday housekeeping practices. Concealed behind walls, care workers' generative labor enables older adults to be praised as living on their own, "independently." These concealments make invisible the forms of inequality and interdependence that make older adults' lives possible.

Independent Living

Housekeeping as Personkeeping

Harriet Cole grudgingly adjusted to life in her apartment in a subsidized senior housing high rise. Its address in the heart of Bronzeville reminded her of the neighborhood's glory days at the center of African American society when she was a young woman. But it was a bit too far from Hyde Park, the elite enclave where her church, her doctors, and her social life were located. She appreciated that the building's entrance was well protected. Before being allowed up the elevator, visitors needed to show their identification to a security guard, who called residents to make sure the visitor was welcome. She also liked that the building offered a full schedule of exercise classes and activities. Mrs. Cole was pleased when the building was remodeled and she was moved to a new apartment from a middle floor to one of the highest floors in the building. She appreciated the security, the view, and the sense of prestige she gained from being so high up. She liked the updated kitchen and the new hallway décor.

Mrs. Cole mourned the many pieces of ornate furniture she had been forced to sell when she moved out of her large home and into a small two-bedroom apartment several years before we met. She treasured the few pieces of her living room set that she had brought with her. She kept them covered in plastic, their presence more decorative than utilitarian. Carefully arranged photographs on a long credenza holding her television depicted Mrs. Cole with her husband, as well as with local celebrities, business elites, and pastors. The latter had once been the primary clients of her insurance business. One frame held the vintage cover of a prominent African American magazine graced by a glamorous portrait of Mrs. Cole from her modeling days.

For all the amenities of the new building, it did not compare to the home she had shared with her husband, with its many rooms, ornate décor, and especially its privacy. Mrs. Cole was suspicious of her new neighbors. She disapproved of their lifestyles, their noisy kin, and their poverty. She refused to get to know any of them, rejecting their invitations and their neighborly requests to borrow a cup of flour. She believed they were largely the kind of people who were slovenly, lazy, and bad at planning for the future. How else had they ended up dependent on government subsidies in their old age? Mrs. Cole disapproved of how some of her neighbors at the senior housing complex lived, because, "some of the senior people are out of touch and some shouldn't be by themselves." She thought they let their family members take advantage of them and did not keep their homes nicely enough.

Mrs. Cole was proud of her remaining possessions and fastidious about how they were cleaned and cared for. She held Virginia Jackson, her home care worker, to exacting housekeeping standards. She wanted her kitchen and bathroom scrubbed twice a week and every surface dusted at least that often. She inspected Virginia's work thoroughly at the end of each visit, pointing out a stray hair remaining in her bathtub or a spot of dust Virginia had overlooked. To continue living independently, she thought that "you should be able to think for yourself and keep yourself and your house well and do the things you got to do." For Mrs. Cole, housekeeping was a way of sustaining independence, and a sign of sustained personhood. She downplayed the ways she relied on Virginia to maintain her home, focusing instead on the many ways she remained in control of her home and life.

This chapter addresses the social relationships that make it possible for older adults to live independently. In home care, the term "housekeeping" takes on a double meaning: both keeping houses clean, and enabling older adults to keep their houses. Home care workers keep houses as a means of keeping independent persons by maintaining materially familiar spaces, reproducing long-standing routines, and by concealing these forms of care. Homes, and the care of homes, play a central role in maintaining older adults' senses of independence in part because of the ways that home care workers' housekeeping labor is hidden. Concealing the care workers' labor maintains the values of independent living and autonomy but makes it difficult to recognize or reward their crucial contributions to older adults' specific lives and to the broader social and economic life of the country. Despite their labor invested in keeping house for others, home care workers often face ongoing housing instability due in part to the lack of economic remuneration and social recognition they receive for their labor.

Housekeeping as Personkeeping

In the United States, where conceptions of personhood are deeply tied to notions of private property, changes to homes and households can feel especially threatening.[1] Home care training videos reflected the widespread idea that living in a private dwelling entitles people to autonomy and self-determination, repeating the common phrase that a person's "home is her castle." Given the importance of living in a private home to cultural understandings of personhood and independence, many older Chicagoans clung to their homes even when doing so meant risking isolation and abandonment. By taking care of houses and making them safe places for older adults to live, home care workers made it possible for older adults to meet cultural expectations of independence.

In diverse places around the world, homes act as extensions of persons, offering a material medium with which to enact techniques of the self and social personhood. Older Chicagoans' emphasis on staying at home as a way of sustaining personhood is one example of the profound connections between houses, persons, and social relations around the world. Anthropologists Janet Carsten and Stephen Hugh-Jones argue that houses, bodies, and minds are "in continuous interaction" and that, as people make homes in their own image, they use them to "construct themselves as individuals and groups."[2] In this way, houses become extensions of persons, simultaneously creating and reflecting their tastes and ways of interacting with others. Caring for houses can thus be a central form of caring for persons and their social relations.

While some older adults continue to inhabit dwellings in which they have lived for much of their adulthoods, others move into places better suited to growing older. In either situation, home care workers play a crucial role in the continued generation of these places as homes, as places that are deeply bound up with the histories, memories, and personalities of their clients. For most of the older adults I knew in Chicago, living at home not only affirmed their continued status as independent persons, it also meant that they had not yet been relegated to widely feared and maligned sites of institutional care. Nursing homes, assisted living facilities, and other group homes for older adults all share the unhappy distinction of being viewed as sites of neglect, abandonment, and social death.[3]

Houses contain and shape intimate social bonds, organizing the lives of their inhabitants, even as changing architectures reflect changing social relations. As a simultaneously stable and dynamic locus of daily life, houses often figure critically in the ways that people contend with social and personal change. Houses create the appearance of permanence, while dynamically reflecting and generating personal, familial, and social change.[4] People persistently alter houses to meet the needs of different moments in their inhabitants' lives, such that houses provide apparent stability even as they are made to accommodate changing gender relations, bodily capacities, and economic circumstances.

In old age, the experiential permanence of houses and household objects often takes on particular significance because of the ways that dwellings become invested with intimate memories, long-standing routines, and dense webs of interwoven meanings and emotions.[5] Even though many older Chicagoans live alone, they live alongside objects that bore the marks of lives shared with others. Homes thus become central resources in older adults' attempts to resist the unmaking of personhood. Home care workers help older adults resist threats to personhood by performing the labor that makes it appear that houses are unchanged even as assistive devices, medications, and the other ephemera of aging in the United States increasingly take up residence in elders' homes.[6] Much in the same way that care workers make subtle adjustments to diets and routines to care for older adults' bodies, they make subtle adjustments to homes to make them safer or more comfortable for older adults while preserving the social and aesthetic organization of the home. Care workers avoided the minor ruptures in daily life that could cause confusion by attending to the smallest details of each home's organization and by honoring the ways that previous members of clients' households continued to shape their organization and routine. As home care workers cared for homes, they generated material continuity and independent personhood in older adults' lives.

For many older Americans, living independently means having control over the rhythms and objects of one's household. It also means feeling self-sufficient. Yet workers' presence in clients' homes often threatens elders' senses of independence. Houses are not simply passive sites for care. Rather, the aesthetic and spatial organization of houses allows and constrains different kinds of activities, structuring the possibilities for care.[7] Older Chicagoans moved around their homes in highly routinized ways, spending time in different rooms according to the time of day. Workers attuned their care to these spatiotemporal routines, alternating between working outside of their clients' view and socializing in the same space as them. Through these creative uses of space, workers and older adults simultaneously removed workers' housekeeping labor from older adults' view and sustained the home as a space of intimate sociality. Older adults were spared the discomfort of witnessing the labor that sustained their households, which helped them feel self-sufficient. Older adults and workers in Chicago also used discursive and racial techniques to conceal workers' presence in older adults' homes. Together, these practices make it appear that older adults are able to keep households on their own. They also make it easier to downplay the crucial generative labor home care workers do to sustain older adults' lives. Obscuring the role workers play in enabling older adults to live independently also conceals the connections between the structures of home care and workers' economic and domestic instability.

Focusing on the independence of older adults makes it appear that the instability of care workers' households is distinct from their paid housekeeping labor, when in practice they are intimately connected. Workers make it possible for older adults to live independently using skills and sensibilities similar to those they use to sustain their own homes. Moreover, older adults depend upon generative labor occurring in workers' households located in distant neighborhoods. There, families collaborate to create households capable of nurturing their inhabitants—including care workers—amid ongoing poverty and instability.

Care workers struggled to live in a manner considered independent due to their limited incomes, unsafe neighborhoods, and ongoing policy changes to Chicago's public housing programs. In the decade prior to my fieldwork, the city of Chicago dismantled its infamous public housing projects, displacing thousands of low-income residents.[8] The upheaval caused by their relocations reverberated through families and neighborhoods for years, as competition for low-income housing increased without a similar uptick in safe housing or subsidies. Many of the workers I knew moved at least once (or were planning to move) during the two years I was in Chicago. Accessing public subsidies for housing could be a demeaning process, as officials probed into the details of applicants' economic, legal, and familial lives. The practices that enable older adults to live independently simultaneously conceal the ways they are embedded in broader structures that generate instability in care workers' households.

"Let Him Get Comfortable"

I never once rang the doorbell or knocked on John Thomas's door over the many months I visited him and Doris. As I drove up to his home, he always stood, posture perfectly straight, waiting in the open door of his midcentury ranch. Located on a block with small suburban lots, evenly cut lawns, and tidy landscaping, Mr. Thomas's home was a model of modest midcentury aesthetic taste. The neighborhood, in a near northern suburb of Chicago, had been home to white middle-class families since at least the 1950s, when the Thomas family moved in. Located just a block from a major freeway in one of the most prestigious and affluent school districts in Chicago, it attracted ever-wealthier families. The high-ceilinged mansions being built nearby were rapidly encroaching on Mr. Thomas's block, leaving him irritated about the ostentatious and discordant additions his next-door neighbors made to their home. Their new second story blocked the sunlight in his single-story home. He was equally irritated by rising property taxes on the home he had lived in for more than 50 years.

When expecting someone, he sat in his blue velour reclining chair located next to the large picture window in his living room. From this comfortable perch, he had a perfect view of the street. He opened the tinted glass door of his stereo cabinet, located under the television, a few feet in front of his chair. Angling the glass so that its dark surface reflected the street behind him, he could keep an eye on cars driving up the street behind him while simultaneously monitoring the clock on his cable box and watching his beloved Weather Channel. This clever arrangement meant he knew as soon as someone parked outside his home. Despite his slow, shuffling steps, he could easily make it to the door to welcome guests.

Visitors entered directly into Mr. Thomas's combined living and dining room. A wood table with four chairs sat just inside the door, with the seating area and television set further inside the room, arranged to provide views of both the picture window and the television. Except for the two matching blue recliners, the furniture all appeared to date from the time Mr. Thomas and his wife purchased the house. Mr. Thomas purchased the recliners after his wife's illness left her homebound, as he wanted somewhere comfortable for her to sit. He had not changed anything in the room since she passed away, though he admitted that the blue floral upholstery and other décor were much more feminine than suited his taste. He still spoke of the home and its inhabitants in the plural, as "our house."

Staying in the house had been painful for Mr. Thomas after his wife died. It was too much house for him. Every object, every surface, reminded him of their 64-year marriage. Yet moving to a smaller apartment or retirement home was unthinkable. Abandoning it would mean abandoning his wife, the home she had so lovingly created for him, and his life as a devoted husband and father. The Thomas family moved to the suburbs from the city when John Jr. was four and had lived there ever since. Moving out would mean fundamentally altering the little habits and routines that connected Mr. Thomas to his past. And Mr. Thomas liked his routines. In more than 40 years of work, he had only been absent unexpectedly once, when he had a heart attack and emergency quadruple bypass surgery in his fifties. He had also only been late to work once in all those decades, despite Chicago's unpredictable traffic, and that was back in the 1970s when a massive snowstorm closed down the freeway. He was an hour late to work that day.

The home was at the center of Mr. Thomas's daily routine. Though it had changed a great deal from his married days, his routine still traversed familiar ground. He had already given up so much. For example, after the bicycle accident that injured his ear, he started riding a stationary bike in the guest room for an hour before dawn. He went to the same restaurant every morning, where he and his wife used to eat regularly. The short drive was the perfect distance to keep up his driving skills, he said, but not so far that it would be dangerous if he got into trouble (he never specified what kind of trouble he was worried about). After breakfast, he went home and watched the Weather Channel. In the mid-afternoon, he drove a few short blocks across the highway to a favorite bar where he had a drink, ate one of their specialty soups—baked potato soup was his favorite—and flirted with the waitresses. He usually ate something light that Doris prepared ahead of time for his supper. Most evenings, Mr. Thomas's next-door neighbors, Linda and Jim Whitting, invited him over for a glass of wine after supper. He sometimes lingered, talking with them for hours. Linda had lived next door for nearly 15 years, through her first marriage and divorce. She spoke of Mr. Thomas as her second father and kept a close eye on him. Without these routines, Mr. Thomas did not know what he would do with his days. Though the house was a source of bittersweet memories, it also anchored him to his previous life, providing material stability as his body and social relationships changed.

Unlike many men of his generation, Mr. Thomas shared housekeeping duties with his wife throughout their marriage. The eldest son of a widowed prison janitor, Mr. Thomas had always helped with cooking and housework and did not see why it should be different when he was married. He saw his more equal partnership with his wife as a sign of his continued independence, since he did not need to rely on her to keep his household functioning. He took some teasing from other men about his unusual approach to marriage but stood his ground. "The people who used to live next door, the guy used to kid me. He said, 'You don't have to do that. Let her do all that.' I said, 'I get a lot of stuff from her that you don't get from your wife. So there's your answer.' My only answer to that is why shouldn't I help when I'm working and she's working too. That's the way I look at it."

When Linda and the social worker at the local senior center first suggested he get a home care worker, Mr. Thomas resisted. He was perfectly capable of taking care of himself and his home without help. But he was losing weight, and he was lonely. When he fell carrying laundry down the steep basement stairs, he finally relented and hired Belltower to provide him with a home care worker. He told me, "It was a little on the tough side because in the first place I didn't figure I needed any help. But now, it breaks up the week with her here 2 days a week. I said I'm hungry so that's when we started going out to eat. That kills an hour and a half or so and we'd come home and she'd start, 'Did you do the bed yet?' or something like that, or she'd do the wash. Later on the next day she'd do the kitchen or run the sweeper. She keeps the house real clean." He continued, "She does things that I think you don't need to, like scrub these kitchen floors every week, you know. I used to do it once a month and the same way with the bathroom. She scrubs it on Monday when she's here and on Friday when she's here." Though Mr. Thomas did not think the house needed to be kept quite so clean, his wife had been fastidious about keeping the house spotless. Doris took her cues from the general tidiness of the house, despite Mr. Thomas's protestations that she cleaned too often. Like other older adults, Mr. Thomas downplayed how much help he needed.

Doris recognized that the home was a source of both stability and pain for Mr. Thomas. She cared for the home with meticulous attention to detail. After returning home from their breakfast, she changed into scrubs, preparing for the sweaty work. If it was laundry day, she started it first thing so that it would be finished and folded before she left that afternoon. Otherwise, Mr. Thomas would try to manage the laundry himself, despite his doctor's repeated exhortations that he should no longer go up and down the steep basement stairs. Next, Doris cleaned the bedroom. She took her time making his bed, making sure the linens lay perfectly flat as she tucked the edges into perfect hospital corners. The bed made, she dusted every surface carefully, lifting each item and replacing it exactly where she found it. When Doris showed me how to do this, she emphasized how important it was to put each item in exactly the same place, especially on Mr. Thomas's night table, since even small changes could mean he would struggle to find things in the night. She gingerly cleaned Mrs. Thomas's nightstand with the same care, noting that it was "sad" and "touching" that Mr. Thomas kept his deceased wife's things sitting at the ready. As she cleaned, Mr. Thomas stayed out of the way, usually sitting on his reclining chair watching the Weather Channel.

Doris kept her home with similar care. She lived in a modest two-bedroom apartment on the second floor of a small apartment building in one of Chicago's far north suburbs. The building was in poor condition, but Doris liked that the neighborhood was quiet and safe. She spent weeks making the basic, somewhat dingy, apartment livable after moving from Wisconsin. She scrubbed every surface with her usual vigor. She sewed colorful curtains out of blackout fabric for the living room and her bedroom to protect her from the sunlight, since it triggered flare-ups of her lupus. She used the extra fabric to make matching pillows and other decorations. When I visited, Doris apologized for the clutter, pointing toward neatly organized shelves of children's toys, explaining that her grandson's things had taken over the apartment. In the kitchen, rows of homemade canned beans and vegetables lined the shelves.

Doris liked her new town, and its location made it easier for her to visit family back in Wisconsin when she had time off. Still, even with normal traffic, it often took her an hour to get to Mr. Thomas's home. When gas prices rose to over $4 a gallon in the summer of 2007, it cost Doris several hours' worth of wages to fill the tank of her 15-year-old Chevy sedan so she could get to work. She wanted to buy a newer car that would get better gas mileage, or perhaps move to an apartment closer in, but she did not know how she would save enough money to do either when she was spending so much of her paycheck just getting to and from work.

Doris brought her housekeeping skills to her work with Mr. Thomas. She wanted to make his home a cheerful place that reflected his personality, much as she had transformed her own apartment. She worried that Mr. Thomas would view any changes as an attempt to eliminate evidence of his wife's influence in the home. When she first started working for Mr. Thomas, she quickly realized that though a number of items in the home were threadbare and needed to be replaced, she would need to make changes gradually. Mr. Thomas was frugal to a fault and resisted making new purchases just for the sake of appearances. Even more important, rapid changes would disrupt Mr. Thomas's sense that his current life was connected to the life he shared with his wife. At the same time, Doris thought it was important to help Mr. Thomas adjust to the changes in his life by making small changes to the home that better reflected his gendered tastes. "You don't make changes right away. You have to let him get comfortable before moving things that was close to him, like a security blanket. Everything that I move or touch belongs to his wife and he and his wife was together for over 60 years and they real close. He visits her [grave] every Sunday."

Doris helped Mr. Thomas alter the home's décor to better reflect its masculine inhabitant by taking on the roles and activities of his deceased wife—reminding him that it was inappropriate to have linens that were falling apart, prodding him to shop for bathmats, sewing him new curtains in her free time. It was precisely by imaginatively inhabiting these typically feminine social and relational roles that she was able to coax him into accepting the changes in his life and reflecting them through changing the materiality of his home. In doing so, she deployed a kind of gendered imagining of what kind of person he should be—one connected to his history as a loving husband and yet not so paralyzed by the loss of that role that he was unable to eat or maintain his home.

Doris described her approach as a series of suggestions that built on even the slightest momentum for change: "So you got to let him move stuff, and once he got started moving, you got to take it slow. You got to suggest things carefully. In the bathroom, when I started suggesting the green rugs. I washed them and all the back of it came loose and I said, 'Oh, Mr. Thomas, we got to go shopping.' I go in and say, 'Your wife had this color. We going to get some new stuff. This is it. We can't wash this no more because it's going to fall apart.' He said, 'My wife used to go to Carsons.' But they closed. He told me about Target, so one day we took time and went to Target and got some new bath rugs."

She continued, describing the process as a kind of emotional choreography. "He would tell me what his wife used to do this and that. . . . Anyway, in order to make that person comfortable and trust you, you got to move when they move. Don't move before. Let them start and once they start, they'll be able to trust you and they are just able to get their changes. You can't go fast, and not a big change. You can't do it BOOM, you got to take it slow." As an example, she described, "when I made him new curtains, it was hard to change because that's what his wife had when she was living. But I said, 'she still lives, she lives in you [Mr. Thomas] and when people come into the house and it's different because the shower curtain got changed, it's okay.' So, I said, 'we're going to redo your bathroom. There's no woman staying here, only thing we got is man's stuff. You don't want no completely pink bathroom. You need blue, or a mix of pink and green. We're going to work on this.' And we're getting there."

Doris described her efforts to update Mr. Thomas's home as a kind of dance that he led while she took on the feminine role. In approaching housekeeping in this manner, she enabled Mr. Thomas to continue to feel like a dutiful husband without being so beholden to his history that he refused all alterations to the space. By moving at his pace, Doris enabled Mr. Thomas to gradually accept the changes to his life without feeling like he was becoming an entirely new person. As Doris increasingly took on wifely aesthetic responsibilities in Mr. Thomas's household, she also became his confidante, providing him with wifely companionship and emotional support.

Doris's efforts extended well beyond her working hours. "When he can't sleep, he calls me. Him being there by himself, he be thinking about his wife and what he went through for years and he just be lonesome. I talk to him: 'Did you check your mail?' He says, 'I did that.' 'Did you check the house and make sure all the doors are locked?' I give him conversation. He loves John Wayne and cowboy pictures. I say, 'get up and go in there and see what's on TV.' He was fussing." Doris's care work followed her back to her home and into the wee hours of the night. She felt it was her moral responsibility to continue caring off the clock. She said, "I worry if I don't do these things he might not live very long. His heart would give out. He has heart problems too. I say the goodest things I could think of as a woman. I put myself in the same place that I am his wife as a woman figure. I won't say anything negative in no kind of way." During these late-night phone calls, Doris coached Mr. Thomas to look after his home and engage in his favorite, overtly masculine entertainments as a way of countering painful memories of the last years of his wife's life. In doing so, she used the familiarity of his masculine and husbandly roles as a way of reminding him of other parts of his life as well as of anchoring him in the mundane pleasures of the present.

As Doris went through the housekeeping tasks that comprised her official job description, she also helped Mr. Thomas adjust to life without his wife. She kept his home tidy and helped him avoid dangerous activities like climbing the stairs. She gently changed the décor to reflect social changes in the household while preserving it as a material connection to Mr. Thomas's earlier life. In her actions, Doris recognized and therefore sustained Mr. Thomas's social personhood. She showed Mr. Thomas that she saw him as still masculine, still exerting control over his home and life. She tended to his home in a way that enabled others to see him in the same light. By keeping his home, altering it very slowly to reflect the changes in his life, she connected his past to his present and enabled him to live in a manner considered independent.

"These Are These People's Houses"

Getting Margee Jefferson back home was a herculean task. Margee tripped and fell one morning while her son Bertram was at work. Bertram lived with her, but he was gone from 7 a.m. until 6 p.m. each weekday, working downtown as a legal clerk. So she lay on the floor for more than seven hours until he returned. After a few days in the hospital while they treated her injured hip, she moved to a nursing home. The emergency medical workers reported that her home was unsafe, and the hospital social worker would not approve her returning home until the home was made safe. Indeed, trip hazards were everywhere, as the home was filled with the collected possessions and detritus of decades of continuous habitation. Her bedroom was up a steep flight of steps, which she could no longer navigate safely. In the upstairs bathroom, the only shower and bathtub in the house were covered with thick green sludge.

Margee and Bertram lived in a large two-story single-family home on Chicago's far west side, in a neighborhood of stately homes. The home had once belonged to Margee's in-laws. Margee and her husband had shared the house with her in-laws for years and raised their two sons and two daughters there. Her husband refused to let her get rid of her in-laws' possessions, even decades after they passed away. The beautiful antique mahogany dining furniture could barely be seen under accumulated objects. Inside the ornate buffet sat Margee's mother's elegant wedding china, which Margee said she had barely ever used because the 14-karat gold edges required hand washing. In the study, the glass floor-to-ceiling bookshelves overflowed with her father-in-law's legal books, while Margee's paperback romance and mystery novels lay in piles on the floor.

Even before she fell, Margee was having a terrible year. Or two years. She wasn't really sure how long it had been since her husband passed away. She lost track of time when she stayed in the nursing home. He had died suddenly. One day he was being admitted to the hospital because of a pain in his abdomen. A few days later he was dead. And then, only a few months later (she thought, but she couldn't be sure), her son Ernest died unexpectedly. He came home from work one evening complaining of a stomachache. Margee remembered in agonizing detail that Ernest had gone upstairs that evening to rest and never came back down.

She wished she had paid more attention to his pain, taken him more seriously. Called an ambulance. But Ernest had always been quiet, never complained much. It was just a stomachache. She still did not know why he died. It had been a terrible, terrible time.

Margee did not mind the nursing home as much as she thought she would because "the food was really good and the care was pretty good. But it wasn't home." She wanted to move home, and badgered her son and daughters repeatedly to figure out a way for her to return home. She was afraid of nursing homes and hospitals, even though she admitted they took good care of her. So that was how she ended up hiring Belltower. Or, more accurately, it was how her daughter, the rich one who lived in California, ended up hiring Belltower.

The agency spent weeks preparing the Jefferson home for Margee's return. When Carmen Rodriguez, the supervisor in charge of the case, first saw the house, she realized she would need to devote an unusual amount of resources to cleaning it in order to make it safe. Carmen realized that the agency might not make much money on the case, but took it anyway, since she believed that "it's a mission we're doing." She brought in two or three home care workers a day—as many as she could spare—to clean out the home. In the first several days, they took 44 bags of trash to the dump and donated more than 80 boxes of books to the local library. It took one worker an entire day to clear out and sanitize the refrigerator. Finally, the downstairs living room, dining room, library, bathroom, and kitchen were decluttered enough that Carmen felt it was safe to move Margee back home. Everyone agreed that Margee could no longer be left home alone, so her daughter paid for a care worker to arrive before Bertram left for work each morning and stay until he returned home in the evening. They installed a hospital bed in one corner of the large living room, eliminating the need for Margee to climb the stairs. Without access to the shower, Carmen decided sponge baths would suffice. Carmen formulated a plan in many stages to clean the remaining areas of home. Margee's home care worker could complete them while Margee napped.

The first care worker that Carmen assigned to Margee did not work out. Carmen wanted Margee on a strict schedule and the first worker had not been able to get Margee to adhere to it. Margee was stubborn. She just ignored her home care worker's directions and did what she pleased. Carmen assigned Grace Washington to the case, hoping that

Grace would be better able to coax Margee into the desired routine. Grace had the gift of being simultaneously firm and encouraging. In the less than three months she had worked with Belltower, she had already proven herself a hard worker, and a fastidious housekeeper.

I met Margee and Grace when Carmen invited me to observe Grace's 90-day employment review. Carmen, Margee, and I sat at Margee's dining room table, large enough to seat at least eight or ten people. Its broad expanse was covered in a freshly laundered and ironed tablecloth, the fine embroidery and starched appearance a stark contrast to the clutter piled on top of the buffet and along the dining room walls. Grace flitted between the dining room and the kitchen, nervously offering us ice water and tidying up the space. Carmen asked Margee how she was doing, how she liked Grace, and if Grace was doing everything she was supposed to. Margee admitted that she resisted most of Grace's efforts, and told us, "Grace does everything I'll let her do. But I was raised to do for myself, and I want to do for myself." Carmen tried to convince Margee to accept more help, telling her, "you've earned a bit of rest. We all hope someone will help us when we need it, and you deserve it. Also, your daughter is paying for you to get this help, and she'll be upset with us if she finds out we're not doing everything we're supposed to." Carmen noted that Grace was doing a good job getting Margee to eat healthier meals. She told Margee that Grace was also evaluated on whether or not Margee soaked her feet every day, so "If you don't let her, it makes Grace look bad." As Carmen spoke, Margee shrugged her shoulders and then stared into space, ignoring Carmen's badgering tone. Grace stared at her feet.

Working in Margee's home was quite a shock for Grace. She lived in a tidy two-bedroom duplex with her husband and granddaughter. Their house was in the far southeast corner of Chicago, where the city curves eastward toward Lake Michigan. Her neighborhood, like many in that part of the city, was full of once middle-class homes that now had peeling paint and frayed awnings. The neighborhood had long since ceased to house middle-class families, the homes now filled by families struggling to get by on incomes from legal low-income employment, under-the-table (meaning not included in official employment and tax rolls) work, and illegal trade. Grace's husband, for example, intermittently worked "off the books" at a friend's auto repair shop. Grace's son had recently left home to attend college in Florida, and her daughter and granddaughter often stayed with Grace.

Like Margee's home, Grace's house was full of possessions, though the similarities ended there. Grace kept her things meticulously clean and organized. Each time I visited, the upholstery of their pristine 1970s living room furniture showed lines from recent vacuuming. Children's toys shared space with sculptural arrangements of televisions from multiple decades. The home was immaculately clean, and Grace kept the dining table permanently set with ornately patterned black- and gold-rimmed china.

Grace and her husband hoped to move soon. They were enrolled in a rent-to-own program through Housing and Urban Development (HUD) that was helping them find a new place. Grace longed for a home in a safer neighborhood, with better access to public transportation. She longed for a shorter commute. The program required them to have a reliable income. They had recently become eligible because Grace worked nearly 50 hours a week with Margee. She normally arose at five o'clock in the morning in order to make it to Margee's home before Bertram left for work at eight.

Grace was grateful for the work, despite the long commute and challenging circumstances. She was proud that her efforts made it possible for Margee to stay at home. Still, she was critical of Carmen's decision to take the case. Grace told me, "This lady [Margee] shouldn't have been allowed to live in that house. That house was unlivable. Where was the social workers? Where was the big bosses? Where was the peoples when they took this case and if Carmen took this case, what the hell was on her mind? What the hell makes them think she can take this case? What if she didn't meet a person like me and didn't care? Then what was going to happen? You still going to go in there and take that lady's money and these people [Margee's children] that are paying big bucks for somebody to come out. You still going to take their case? What if you didn't have a person like me?" Grace suggested that it was only her particular commitments to care, learned among kin, that enabled her to withstand and improve the difficult circumstances in which she was asked to care.

Though Grace suspected the agency's reasons for taking the case were monetary rather than moral, Grace was committed to doing what she could to improve her client's life. She told me, "Still, no one should live like this, and [Margee's] just an old woman. So I'm okay working here and cleaning it up. I'm not gonna touch that upstairs bathroom though. It's too dirty, a professional should do it. It's not like I've got insurance if I get sick from working in there. Then I'd miss work and where would I be?" In suggesting that a professional should clean the moldy bathroom, Grace was critiquing her own lack of institutional support and protection. For all the relational boundaries home care agencies tried to create between workers' and older adults' households, Grace's fear of transmitting infection between the two homes reveals the ways that the structures of home care work inadequately protect care workers' vulnerable bodies and their economically precarious households.

It was difficult for Grace to understand how Margee and Bertram lived. When she arrived at the home each Monday morning, she'd find four or five overflowing trash bags piled near the back door. Showing them to me, she said, "How come he [Bertram] leave them there? How hard is it to walk them to the cans behind the garage?" She'd also find soiled adult diapers lying on the bathroom floor, and Margee's underwear left lying where they fell. She compared the domestic habits instilled in her by kin with those of her clients: "They just nasty, dirty people. They maybe always been this way, they don't even seem to mind or notice that it's filthy. As soon as no one's there to clean up after them, the house be filthy again. The way I was raised, a strict black family and all that, if you had two shirts, you washed one while you wore the other. Even if you had to wash every day." Through this comparison, Grace highlighted the ways that wealthier households came to depend on the strict hygiene of working-class black households like her own.

Despite these differences, Grace's approach to caring for Margee and the Jefferson home was inspired by her care for her own household and kin. She strove to make her home a place of comfort and happiness. She told me, "I love cooking big dinners on holidays. I tell everyone, 'Look, you all come to my house, you have to take your shoes off. Just bring your appetite and bring your laughing because we gonna laugh and have a good time. If you got an attitude, you stay outside of my door.'" She continued, "You coming into my house, you coming into a happy house. You want to come into a house where you can sit and feel comfortable." This was linked to her desire to create a home different from the violence of her childhood. "I said that if I would ever get grown up and got my own place and anybody come to my house, I never going to have anybody feel uncomfortable or scared to get up to go to the bathroom or scared to ask for something. Make yourself at home. Do what you do."

Grace imagined her household expansively, extending her care from her own home to her mother's home and her client's home. In each space, she strove to create an atmosphere that was equally clean and comfortable. "I noticed that like on holidays when we used to go to my mom's house, after I started having children, my sisters would come over and I would be so mad because they would come over on the holidays and they would tear up my mama's house so bad. I would never leave until my mama's house was that clean and my mama didn't have to do nothing. My mama would tell you that right today." As "a home-knitted person," Grace continually strove to keep the things and people who comprised her household together, safe, and happy.

Grace brought a similar domestic sensibility to her care work, wanting her clients to feel comfortable in their own homes. This was particularly challenging at Margee's home given the drastic changes that had been made to make it safe. When Grace first arrived, she immediately wanted to help Margee because she thought, "how would I feel if my grandparent would be living like this? I would be devastated and it immediately touched my heart. . . . I had to call for the gloves and to get the stuff to keep me sanitized and to keep me from getting sick. Any other person in their right mind would say, 'Hell, with this job. Hell, I ain't taking this shit. This is a God damn garbage place.' This is no damn house. This is a place where you come and throw garbage because that's how bad the house looks." Although Grace did not think it was appropriate for a company to send its employees to work in a filthy, dangerous environment, she agreed to take the job. Sure, she needed a steady income to qualify for the HUD rent-to-own program that would stabilize her own household. But money was not the primary reason she worked so diligently to transform Margee's home. She argued that her wages were too low to motivate her dedication, saying, "When I go in there, it's definitely not about the money because the money ain't all that. I don't get into this because of the salary. I get into this because what I feel in my heart. I have a senior mother. I have a senior father."

Grace used the same language to describe caring for Margee's home and her own household, moving seamlessly between describing improvements in the house and improvements in Margee's mood. "Mind you, in a week's time, that house was livable, clean, and sanitized. You can walk through there and you can take a dust test and you couldn't find a thing. When I got there, [Margee] was in such a depressing stage. She wouldn't talk. I just found a way to get around. I'm like a persistent person. When you say don't, I say do. When you say can't, I say can. I'm sorry, that's just me." Grace continued, "I'm not going to let you sit here and be depressed and wallow in your misery because, yes, you have lost loved ones. We all have lost loved ones but we're still here. We got to move on. We got to live. Life is still happy and fun and life is all what you make it. As long as I got to be here, I'm going to make you happy. I'm going to make sure you are alright and I'm going to do things. You got to do things in steps and measures."

For Grace, caring for the home and the people who lived in it were one and the same. "I'm just a neat person. I like a clean house. If I got to be here for 10 hours, hell, it's got to be livable for me. I'm sorry. I can't sit here for 10 hours and I got to step over and I'm scared to go to the bathroom and stuff like that. I can't do that so I got to make this house livable and comfortable for me and for this lady as if this lady is my own grandmother."

Over the months that Grace worked with Margee, Grace's conflicts with Carmen escalated. Initially, she considered Grace one of the agency's best workers. Deeply impressed with the vigor and dedication with which Grace had tackled each gargantuan task in Margee's home, Carmen suggested that they become one of the pairs I focused my research on. As the weeks and months passed, Carmen and Grace butted heads more and more often. Even though Grace was critical of Margee's lifestyle, she believed the older woman had a right to live as she chose in her own home. Grace refused to force Margee into a new routine and insisted on making some changes to the home more gradually. She was concerned about how such radical alterations would affect Margee's well-being. "You can't go in here and go in these people's houses and think yeah you want to make the senior care better. Yeah, you can make it better but you can't go in there and change all the rules." Grace's voice grew louder as she spoke, "This is the people's houses we are talking about and you can't go in there in these people's houses and tell them where we got company policy. Yeah, we got company policy but God damn it, these are these people's houses. You can't go in there and tell these people while these people are paying you their hard-earned money to come here and help them." By now, Grace was nearly yelling as she clearly articulated her moral approach to care. "They are not saying change them. They are saying they need a little bit of help. . . . Now you might have a problem and yes, we can deal with those problems, but you cannot go into these people's houses and change these people's lives according to your standard." Grace argued that clients did not pay Belltower to change their lives, but rather to sustain their ways of life. Grace implicitly endorsed the idea that paying for services entitled people to control how that service was provided. People had the right to determine what happened within their own home whether or not that conformed to the agency's policies. Grace resisted Carmen's instructions to protect Margee's autonomy, an autonomy Grace understood as engendered in part by Margee's continued residence in her home.

The trick, Grace told me, was to make gradual modifications to people's routines rather than drastically upending their ways of life. "That's the main problem that I have with the boss lady, Carmen, because she has a double standard. You cannot change these people's lifestyle. This lady [Margee] is used to doing stuff a certain way. Yes, we can modify it. We can do it a little bit but don't do it so much whereas it's becoming a problem. I was doing it to a way whereas it was working. She was happy. She sits in there and talks to me [for] hours. I don't care if she's telling me the same thing over and over. It doesn't matter. I understand that. To better serve these people, you got to find a way to also keep it by the guidelines, also to keep it by company policy but also try to modify it whereas you are not totally changing these people's lives because you can't go in there and change these people's lives."

To sustain life, Grace believed in sustaining elders' ways of living. Margee's way of life disgusted Grace, yet she accepted that Margee had the right to determine what happened in her own home. While Grace questioned the appropriateness of assigning workers to a dangerous environment, she affirmed Margee's status as an independent person with the right to determine how she lived in her own home. Changes necessary to maintain Margee's health or improve her quality of life should be made gradually and with caution. Despite her concerns, Grace devoted herself to caring for Margee's home as a way of caring for Margee and sustaining her personhood.

Concealing Care

For older adults to be recognized by both themselves and others as independent persons, they not only have to continue to live in a familiar manner, they also have to appear self-sufficient. Workers, older adults, and sometimes agency personnel engage in a number of discursive, spatial, and racial practices that conceal the traces of workers' labor, and which are simultaneously signs of elders' increasing need for help. Some of these techniques work to hide home care workers' labor in plain sight, while other practices work a kind of social alchemy, making home care workers appear as companions or traditional domestic servants.

For example, Mrs. Cole downplayed her reliance on Virginia Jackson. Mrs. Cole asserted that despite receiving home care, she was still able to care for her home and her body with equal vigilance. She asserted that this was proof that she still had "that sense of independence you have to have. I still go to church on Sundays. I still do my bath. I wash my own dishes and I make my bed when I get up. These things have got to be done." Whether or not Virginia came to her home, Mrs. Cole claimed that she would be able to maintain her household because she was able to think clearly and take care of herself. In order to assert that she remained independent after a debilitating stroke, Mrs. Cole discursively erased Virginia's labor and the contributions Virginia made to the maintenance of her household.

Because Mrs. Cole did not acknowledge her reliance on Virginia, she also could not acknowledge that the structures of care upon which she relied were dependent on workers' low wages. Even as Virginia's labor made it possible for Mrs. Cole to continue living independently in her home, Mrs. Cole was critical of Virginia for working a job that could not provide her with financial security and independence. She argued that working for low wages was a form of self-sabotage that showed a lack of self-respect and dangerous willingness to be dependent on others. "If you don't push for something, what are you going to do? One of these days she's going to go around and Social Security's going to be coming up and she won't have none. . . . you got to want something, you know. . . . You got to have a little respect for you and want for yourself." She chalked this up to Virginia's lack of ambition, not considering other factors that might make it difficult for Virginia to find better paying work.

While Virginia's care generated stability and continuity in her clients' households, her own household was unstable. That winter, she was forced to move to a smaller apartment because her landlord raised her rent. Virginia tried to put a brave spin on the move, noting that her new neighborhood had a better reputation than her old one. Still, it was a small third-floor walk-up and was farther from public transportation than her old apartment. Virginia spoke about wanting to find a better job, but she did not have the time to fill out applications and go on interviews, much less to undertake the training she would need to qualify for a better paying position.

Every older adult that I interviewed told me that one crucial component of "good care" was that the worker "just knew" what needed to be done in their home. For older adults, constantly describing each detail of how they like their home kept or meals cooked means announcing their lack of self-sufficiency over and over. When done with great skill and tact, workers' embodied care, such as that described in the previous chapter, helps older adults appear self-sufficient because it enables workers to sustain their clients' ways of life without requiring ongoing instructions from older adults. This makes it possible for older adults like Mrs. Cole and Margee to deny that they need help and emphasizes how much they can do for themselves. In each denial, older adults simultaneously present themselves as still independent and discursively erase the crucial role home care workers play in their lives.

Mr. Sampson particularly appreciated that Kim managed to keep his home tidy without constant instruction because, "someone who comes is super because you get to talk to someone and let them do what is supposed to be done. With Kim, there's nothing I got to tell her to do." Though what was "supposed to be done" intimately involved Mr. Sampson, he spoke as though he had no agency or role in care except to get out of the way. Because Kim was able to work without instruction, Mr. Sampson was able to describe her as a friend he could talk to and who helped out around the house, rather than someone on whom he depended.

Mrs. Silverman's family had employed domestic workers since she was a young child. From these experiences, she learned to treat domestic workers as members of the household. She told me, "You have to treat them like a human being. That's it in a nutshell. You don't put aside food—this is for you and this is for the rest of us. You leave the food in the refrigerator and help yourself. They were just polite to the help.

Never a cross word. They could keep help a long time and enjoyed the help and got along well. Black, white, it didn't matter to them. They really treated the help properly."[9] Mrs. Silverman continued her family's tradition, for example by insisting on paying for Maria's meal at McDonald's when they ate out. For Mrs. Silverman, one way to treat a worker like a human being was to include the worker in some of the shared resources of the household. At the same time, Mrs. Silverman preferred workers who "have a little direction of their own. I can't say, 'Do this, do that.' I make it sound like God knows what you are expecting. If they do it themselves, they do it." Mrs. Silverman's well-intentioned and often kind-hearted efforts to include Maria in her household, combined with her preference for workers who did not require ongoing instruction, worked to obscure Maria's status as an employee whose membership in her household was conditional on pleasing her employer. These language practices thereby helped to sustain the impression that older adults continued to live unchanged and independent lives.

Workers' and older adults' spatial practices also obscured many of the concrete ways that workers contributed to maintaining older adults' households and ways of life, leaving behind the illusion that homes remained perpetually clean and orderly. Every older adult I knew had a preferred chair to sit on in their living or dining room—usually reading or watching television—while workers moved around other parts of the home, cleaning, cooking, and doing laundry. While in the home, workers and older adults were typically only in the same room when eating together, chatting, or conducting personal care like bathing and toileting. Several older adults actually moved from one room in the home to another to maintain this spatial distance while their worker was cleaning the room in which they normally sat. Older adults sometimes described this spatial separation as "staying out of the way," and making sure the worker didn't feel like they were watched and distrusted. Yet this separation also meant that older adults did not see workers performing much of the labor that sustained their ways of life. These spatial practices, much like embodied care and verbal denials of need, helped older adults avoid experiencing themselves as dependent on workers' care, and therefore sustained their senses of independence.

Workers' racial or ethnic background and gender sometimes helped to conceal home care workers, hiding older adults' dependence on workers in plain sight. This was particularly common among Belltower clients. In several cases, white clients who had domestic workers like housekeepers or nannies in their homes earlier in life were more comfortable with black American home care workers. These clients tended to refer to workers as "the help" or "my girl," labels long used in the United States to refer to poor and usually non-white domestic servants. Such terms are widely considered derogatory by both domestic and home care workers. These gendered and racialized naming practices transform home care workers into generic domestic servants, disguising the particular age- and disability-related impetus behind home care workers' labor.

In some cases, older adults avoided hiring workers whose ethnicities might reveal their need for care. Supervisors at Belltower reported that a surprising number of clients refused Filipina care workers even though Filipinas were widely stereotyped as excellent, highly trained care providers. Supervisors told me that these elders worried that employing a Filipina worker would be unmistakable proof that they needed significant amounts of care, not just help around the house.

In some cases, older adults preferred workers of the same racial background as themselves, not because of explicit racism but because the racial similarity would better disguise the worker. For example, Celia Tomas told me about one Belltower client whose children had hired the agency because their mother was experiencing the early stages of dementia. This woman, who was white, refused multiple care workers, insisting that she did not need help. She was mortified that her friends would learn she could not manage her apartment anymore. Eventually, Celia matched her with a worker who was also white. A few months later, the client proudly took the worker along on her daily walks, introducing the worker to neighbors as a dear and loyal friend. The client so deeply believed that her worker was simply a very helpful friend and not a paid employee that Celia struggled to explain her own periodic phone calls and visits to monitor the worker. Celia, typically forthright about naming racism when she saw it, argued that this client's preference for a white worker had less to do with outright prejudice and more to do with the visibility of a non-white worker in the client's predominantly white neighborhood. Indeed, in that neighborhood, the racial and gender similarities between worker and client helped the worker blend into the scenery. As a white woman, the worker was able to become an unmarked and unremarkable presence in her client's life, hiding her client's growing dependence.

Within the walls of private homes, racial, spatial, and discursive practices obscure the contributions workers make to older adults' households. These concealments capitalize on and exacerbate broader, intersecting structures of racial, gender, and class inequality endemic to the home care industry. Practices that conceal the contributions home care workers make to the lives of their elderly clients through their profoundly empathic skill simultaneously sustain older adults as recognizably independent persons. These concealments also contribute to popular depictions of care workers as unskilled and deserving of only low wages. Together, these concealments threaten workers' social personhood, frequently leaving them reliant on welfare benefits to supplement their incomes and thus portrayed as dependent on the social safety net rather than as crucial contributors to it.

The home care industry exists to enable independent living among older adults. Disability and elder rights activists promote independent living as a civil right that protects the personhood of vulnerable individuals. Policy makers also favor independent living because it reduces the public costs of care since elders remain responsible for their own housing and food expenses. Older adults also favor living at home, amid familiar surroundings. Home care workers make it possible for older adults to live in a manner considered independent by preserving familiar ways of life, sustaining their routines, and keeping their homes. Yet workers and older adults also collaborate in practices that effectively obscure the workers' roles, preserving the experience of self-sufficiency so central to older adults' senses of independence. As workers stabilize the households of their elderly clients, their low wages and long hours contribute to ongoing instability in their own households.

Ongoing instabilities can threaten workers' ability to keep their jobs, manifesting in endemically high levels of worker turnover across the home care industry. The very practices that sustain older adults as independent persons undermine workers' stability, eventually creating insecurity in the lives of workers and older adults alike. In the next chapter, I examine two situations in which care policies and practices that treat older adults and care workers as independent failed to support the profound interdependence that binds together the fates of care workers, older adults, and the families of each.

6

Care Falls Apart

Turnover and the Limits of Independence

Mrs. Silverman spoke rapidly into the telephone, her voice agitated and anxious. "Do you know where Maria is? Do you know why she hasn't called me? She's not coming to work today. Do you know when she will come back?" I had no answers for Mrs. Silverman. She suspected Kathy Hirschorn, the supervisor at Belltower, was withholding information from her. Maybe I would be more forthcoming. It was a frigid Tuesday morning in February, and Mrs. Silverman had been without help since late the previous week, when Maria missed her Friday appointment. Kathy told her that Maria had injured her knee, but Mrs. Silverman thought something else was going on. Mrs. Silverman said that when she spoke to Maria later that Friday, Maria was laughing and joking. She did not sound like a woman in pain. Of course, one of Maria's mantras was to always "show 100%" with her clients, concealing her suffering behind her megawatt smile.

The previous Friday, Mrs. Silverman complained that Maria's absence made it difficult for her to prepare for her son Chip's monthly visit. As soon as she awoke that morning, she stripped the sheets off of her bed and gathered her laundry, anticipating Maria's arrival. She learned a few hours later that Maria would not be coming to work, but refused Kathy's offer for a substitute worker. It would be exhausting to explain to a stranger all the things that needed to be done around the house. And explaining her needs made her feel like she was asking for help, which she hated doing. When Maria started working with her, "she just came right in and knew what to do." How would she get to the grocery store to purchase Chip's favorite egg salad? Who would make his bed? When I offered to help do laundry and put the sheets back on the bed, Mrs. Silverman refused. Eventually, Mrs. Silverman agreed to let her daughter, Susan, take her grocery shopping, but still refused her daughter's offer to help with the rest of the housework. By the time she called me on Tuesday, she was growing desperate. Without Maria's visit, the guest bed sheets would remain unwashed, the house unclean. But Mrs. Silverman did not know how she was going to get her house back in order without Maria. Accepting help from her daughter or from me felt dependent. Paying workers to help with housework, on the other hand, only felt dependent if they had to be told what to do all the time.

Maria was missing work more and more frequently, according to Mrs. Silverman. Each time, Belltower supervisors offered a reasonable explanation. Mrs. Silverman suspected they were excuses. She thought Maria's absences were caused by stress and depression. Maria did not tell Mrs. Silverman many details about her life, but she said enough that Mrs. Silverman knew Maria was having a hard time. She knew Maria was upset that her husband left her without warning. She also knew Maria could not afford her apartment on her own income and was trying to find another place to live. She wondered if Maria's supervisors were aware, if they could do anything to help. Mrs. Silverman worried that after being abandoned by her husband, Maria might leave her job—deserting Mrs. Silverman in the process.

When I spoke with Kathy later Tuesday afternoon, she confirmed that Maria had fallen and aggravated an old knee injury that had never fully healed. She only shared with Mrs. Silverman the vaguest details about Maria's injury because "we did not want to discuss the accident with Mrs. Silverman and get her more worried. We reassured her that all is well and Maria will be there with her on Friday." Kathy, and Belltower, had multiple motivations for assuaging Mrs. Silverman's anxiety. Kathy marketed Belltower as relieving older adults of the emotional and practical consequences of acting as employers. This included worrying about when an injured employee might be able to resume her duties. From Kathy's perspective, Mrs. Silverman's anxiety threatened the durability of her pairing with Maria. If Mrs. Silverman came to feel she could not rely on Maria, she might insist on changing workers, or worse, agencies. With a limited supply of available and suitable workers, it was in the agency's best interest to sustain workable pairings for as long as possible.

Unbeknownst to Kathy, Mrs. Silverman and Maria had exchanged phone numbers many months prior, and Mrs. Silverman's anxiety was exacerbated when Maria did not return several of her phone calls over the weekend. Home care agencies typically discourage (or prohibit) older adults and workers from exchanging telephone numbers, preferring that all communication between the two be mediated by the agency. I was told that this rule protected both workers and older adults from making requests of one another (for example, requesting schedule changes or extra work) that were difficult to refuse. The Belltower employee manual also prohibited workers from "discussing personal problems" with their clients. Together these rules were meant to protect workers and older adults from sharing information with one another, or becoming "too close" in ways that might cause clients to lose confidence in their worker. Indeed, had Mrs. Silverman and Maria followed these rules and allowed the agency to mediate their communication, Mrs. Silverman might have been spared anxiety and doubt. Yet this flow of information also enabled Mrs. Silverman to care for Maria. Through this care and concern, Mrs. Silverman presented herself as a considerate person enmeshed in reciprocal relations, rather than as a vulnerable elder in need of protection.

Maria's absence highlighted the ways that instability in workers' lives was intertwined with instability in elders' lives. As far as I know, Maria continued to work with Mrs. Silverman after I finished fieldwork. Yet for several weeks, the durability of their pairing was threatened by Maria's injury and domestic instability. Even this brief disruption of service panicked Mrs. Silverman. She feared that without Maria she would be unable to sustain the independent lifestyle to which she was accustomed. As Maria's absences revealed, workers' bodily and familial distress hindered their ability to provide the deeply embodied care that sustained elders' independence.

This episode underscored how home care practices and policies that define older adults and workers as separate, independent persons contribute to the home care industry's endemically high turnover rates. By the time I finished fieldwork, three of the home care workers I knew best had quit or were fired. Given that turnover rates in the industry are estimated around 50 percent per year, it is not entirely surprising that turnover among the workers I knew was so high.[1] When I was recruiting worker-client pairs to participate in fieldwork, agency supervisors were inclined to recommend workers they thought were stable and good at their jobs. For this reason, I did not expect that so many of them would no longer be employed by their agencies at the end of fieldwork.

High rates of turnover among this relatively select group suggest that a worker's apparent skill and dedication are not enough to keep them in home care jobs.

Drawing on cases of turnover that occurred during my fieldwork, this chapter examines the ways that home care relationships were destabilized by policies and practices that treat workers and older adults as independent by restricting or penalizing forms of mutuality that sustain their relationships. In some of these cases, other causes of turnover became apparent, for example when workers stole from their clients or when supervisors fired workers with whom they did not get along. Nevertheless, the industry's astronomical turnover rates and perpetual worker shortages require looking beyond individual bad actors to understand how the moral and material structure of home care itself perpetuates instability.

Other studies show that low wages, lack of benefits, lack of opportunity for career advancement, and lack of support are likely causes of high turnover.[2] These factors played a role in each of the cases I observed. With low wages, limited benefits, and minimal welfare support, it is not surprising that the ongoing instability of workers' households often made it impossible for workers to consistently provide the intensive, embodied care they and their clients valued. Complementing these material factors is a broader story of an industry that makes a profit by treating workers as independent persons and lone actors, compensated only for accomplishing tasks specified by formal care plans. The industry thus ignores—and fails to compensate—the intimate relationships that workers forge with older adults and the ways these relationships are sustained by workers' wider webs of kin.

Approaching turnover through the lens of generative labor directs attention to the ways that home care practices meant to sustain lives and persons simultaneously create unequal and unsustainable social relations. Home care workers generate the independent lives of their elderly clients through everyday labor practices that simultaneously forge moral and material bonds between them. Home care practices and agency policies constrain these relationships by limiting flows of knowledge, sentiment, and resources between workers' and elders' households. In the process, home care policy and practice simultaneously envision and constitute workers and older adults as separate, independent persons.

Home care agency policy and practice also generate older adults as independent persons by disregarding workers' embeddedness within under-resourced kin networks. This obscures the profound ways that older adults' and workers' bodies, lives, and households are bound together. These policies and practices thus frame workers' family relationships as external to paid care relationships, even though support from workers' families often made their labor possible.

Knowledge, resources, and obligation circulate between workers' and older adults' households. However, it is workers alone who are penalized when these flows go awry. In seeking to limit flows between clients' households and workers' households, agency and industry policies create conflicts between workers' paid care and care for kin. This hinders workers' abilities to simultaneously care for clients and meet their familial obligations as members of mutually reliant webs of care. From this vantage point, home care is both generative and extractive, as workers are expected to transfer skills and moral understandings developed to care for kin to sustain the lives of paying clients.

Only by conceiving of workers as independent from broader networks of care can workers who miss work to care for their kin be fired for having "too much going on" to be reliable. Only by understanding workers' bodies as disconnected from those of their clients can their exhaustion be reinterpreted as inadequate dedication to their work. Only by imagining workers' lives as separate from those of their elderly clients can reciprocal exchanges be recast as thefts that unscrupulous workers perpetrate on vulnerable elders. It is through the frame of independence that workers' periodic job loss is seen only as a problem for them and their families to cope with. Instead, the home care industry's high rate of turnover should be read as a devastating symptom of the basic contradictions at the heart of home care. Turnover reveals the unsustainability of generating independent persons by exploiting the bodily and relational interconnectedness that sustains human life. Cases of turnover thus raise critical questions about how to create sustainable structures for elder care and other forms of generative labor in the United States.

Dangerous Gifts

Home care agencies prohibit unsanctioned exchanges between workers and older adults.[3] These policies aim to limit relational and material interdependence between workers and older adults. And yet, gift exchanges proliferate in home care relationships. Gifts materially facilitate the complex entanglements and interdependencies that develop between home care workers and older adults. They pose problems in US home care partly because home care agencies and the public at large take what sociologist Viviana Zelizer critiques as a "hostile worlds" approach to questions about the relationship between money and love. Zelizer argues that normative Euro-American moralities imagine that economic markets and intimate life should be kept strictly separate because the norms and goals of each sphere have the potential to pollute and distort those of the other.[4] Cases like home care make visible the flaws in hostile worlds arguments because they show that intimacy and economy are always intertwined in the generation of human lives. People constantly negotiate how to arrange intimate economic relations through everyday practices like gift exchange.

Gift exchange is one of the few forms of social practice that seems to be present in human societies across time and space. Often, people engage in reciprocal exchange as a way of solidifying and extending social relationships through time. Gifts propagate themselves, creating moral expectations for their eventual—rather than immediate—return. It is not surprising, then, that gift exchanges proliferate within capitalist endeavors like home care, coexisting and intertwined with forms of market exchange. Market exchange is distinguished by its immediacy and the calculability of the exchange—market trades do not necessarily create ongoing obligation. The reciprocities generated by gift exchange can also assuage tensions caused by inequality.[5] Home care agencies ban gifts between worker and clients in part because gifts generate moral demands that exceed the agreed upon exchange of wages for care labor.

In the United States, reciprocal exchanges also establish participants as independent persons with the ability to participate in moral relationships.[6] Older adults often reciprocate the care they receive through gifts of money, time, and household goods. Through such exchanges, older adults affirm themselves as socially and morally able, independent persons. Home care agencies' restrictions against gift exchanges thus threaten both elders' personhood and their ability to participate in moral relationships.

Gift exchanges are risky for workers and care relationships, because (as is true for gifts generally) they create expectations and demand reciprocity. The consequences of unreciprocated gifts in home care are doubly risky, as they can be reinterpreted as thefts. Some of the illicit gifts, loans, and favors that clients gave workers were eventually discovered by the agency. This most often occurred when workers failed to meet older adults' expectations for reciprocity and usually lead to the worker's termination. Redefining these exchanges as theft shows that workers alone are held responsible for the consequences of not maintaining professional boundaries between themselves and their clients.

John Thomas and Doris Robinson's relationship was destroyed by this form of ruptured reciprocity. Several months after I completed my fieldwork with Mr. Thomas and Doris, I received a phone call from Mr. Thomas's next-door neighbor, Linda. She thought I would want to know that Mr. Thomas fell at his home a few weeks earlier, injuring himself seriously enough to be hospitalized. By the time Linda called, he was in stable condition, recovering at a luxury nursing home a few minutes from their street. I asked after Doris. Linda was surprised that I hadn't heard the news. Doris had recently been fired for stealing upwards of $13,000 from Mr. Thomas. I was shocked. Unbidden tears welling, shivers of concern coursed through me as I listened to Linda's account of what had happened.

When Mr. Thomas was hospitalized, Linda offered to bring Mr. Thomas his bills and financial records. Sorting through his paperwork, she found a slip of paper on which Mr. Thomas had written only dates and dollar figures. This aroused Linda's curiosity. Mr. Thomas was proud of his meticulous financial record keeping. He had shown me his records, carefully organized in a tall stack of identical leather-bound accounting ledgers. In them he had handwritten every deposit, payment, and purchase he or his wife made since the day they were married. It seemed odd to Linda that he would keep a record of monetary activity anywhere else, much less a random piece of paper. When Linda confronted Mr. Thomas about the slip of paper, he dismissed her concern and refused to tell her what the numbers meant. It was none of her business. Linda persisted for weeks before Mr. Thomas admitted to loaning Doris money. He made Linda promise not to report the transactions to Belltower.

When I visited Mr. Thomas in the nursing home a few days after Linda's call, he told me his version of the story, and how Linda eventually convinced him to report the loans to Belltower. He loaned Doris the money because he had been concerned about her. The first time, she had needed money to get her car repaired so she could make it to work more reliably. She had been consistently late for several months because her car would overheat on the freeway if she forgot to add water to the radiator before she left home. The next time, she could not afford the co-pays on her grandson's glasses and medications. And so it went.

Doris told Mr. Thomas she could not get more work and was having trouble paying the bills. As far as I know, Doris never told Mr. Thomas about her lupus or that she received Social Security disability insurance. Perhaps she concealed her illness and disability status out of a sense of privacy, or because she was hiding her use of government benefits. Perhaps she felt she was protecting Mr. Thomas from worrying more about her than he already did. Perhaps she concealed these aspects of her life in an attempt to follow Belltower's mandate that workers not reveal too much about their personal lives. Whatever her motives, Mr. Thomas did not know that disability benefits and illness limited the number of hours Doris was able to work.

The money Mr. Thomas loaned Doris was money he kept as cash in his safe at home. He kept this money separate from the rest of his savings because he had received it as the proceeds from the sale of his wife's family property. He did not consider it right to spend the money on himself, since he had not earned it. He felt little obligation to pass the money along to his son, a computer engineer who had become wealthy enough to retire by his early fifties. Unconcerned about preserving this part of his estate for descendants, Mr. Thomas saw no reason not to loan some of this money to Doris. It had seemed like the right thing to do. At the same time, he decided that the money in the safe was all he could ethically lend her, since he had to stretch his savings to pay for any care he would need. It would not be right to loan more money and later risk relying on his son to pay for care if he ran out of funds. Though he had taken Doris at her word that she would repay the loans, initially he did not feel comfortable pushing her to do so. They never discussed a repayment schedule. When I asked if he had ever been concerned that Doris might never be able to pay back the loans, he simply shrugged.

A few weeks after Linda found out about the loans, she managed to change Mr. Thomas's mind about reporting them to Belltower. Linda persisted in arguing that it was unethical for him not to report them, worried that Doris might take advantage of other vulnerable older adults. At some point, Mr. Thomas learned that Belltower had previously offered Doris more hours of work, which she declined. He felt lied to and betrayed, and finally agreed to report the loans to Belltower supervisors. Immediately after Mr. Thomas reported the loans, Belltower fired Doris for stealing from Mr. Thomas. Soon after, criminal charges were filed against her and the agency's insurance company filed a civil suit. Belltower's insurance company repaid Mr. Thomas half of the loan amount. It would pay the remainder after they collected from Doris. Through this process, the loans, which Mr. Thomas viewed as almost-gifts, were officially transformed into thefts. With theft on her criminal record, Doris would likely find it difficult to work in a formal elder-care setting again.

When I visited Mr. Thomas in the nursing home, he was visibly upset that he felt he had to report Doris. He worried about her well-being, asking if I knew how she was doing. Still confined to a bed recovering from his fall many weeks before, Mr. Thomas was embarrassed and defensive as he related the whole story to me. He did not want me to think of him as a vulnerable old man who had been duped and taken advantage of. He told me repeatedly that "I knew what I was doing" loaning Doris money, and he still thought it had been the right thing to do. It was the least he could do, and it was a fair trade, since Doris did so much to help him. She regularly did more for him than the tasks listed on his care plan. She updated his bathroom, decorated his house for Christmas, attended his birthday party, and stayed after work to accompany him to his favorite bar for a bite nearly every week. From Mr. Thomas's point of view, he was the more powerful and privileged person in his relationship with Doris, and it was his moral prerogative to help her.

At first glance, this story confirms many people's worst fears about home care. This tale could be easily interpreted as that of a greedy and unscrupulous home care worker playing on the sympathies of a vulnerable older adult who had worked hard his whole life to save for a comfortable retirement. That is not how Mr. Thomas wanted his story told. Mr. Thomas did not think that his need for help around the house rendered him inherently vulnerable or dependent; he did not see himself as someone who had been preyed upon. Rather, Mr. Thomas viewed himself as a caring and generous man with resources and money to spare. Mr. Thomas interpreted what had happened with Doris as a story of reciprocal care and goodwill, eventually compromised when she betrayed his trust.

The unraveling of Mr. Thomas and Doris's relationship is one example of the ways entanglements between workers and older adults run up against policies that imagine older adults and workers as separate entities and ignore their complex interdependence. Home care agency policies imagine care as flowing unidirectionally from worker to client, compensated fully by the wages workers are paid. Through their care for one another, Mr. Thomas and Doris saw their lives as more deeply intertwined than a simple exchange of wages for care labor. For them, care included both the embodied empathy and practical tasks that Doris provided for Mr. Thomas, and genuine concern and economic assistance that Mr. Thomas reciprocally offered Doris. When these entanglements unraveled, Doris alone was held responsible for the ways in which these entanglements violated the clear boundaries required by agencies.

During my fieldwork, many of the exchanges that came to be seen as thefts occurred within a context of ongoing, open, and seemingly voluntary exchanges between workers and older adults. Many older adults' experiences of care were entwined with their experiences of kinship, and their ethical understandings of care suggested that care could not be fully reciprocated by wages. To balance the exchange, older adults proffered money, hand-me-down clothing, and household goods. More frequently, older adults gave their workers paid time off by signing time sheets indicating that workers had worked their assigned hours, despite tardiness or early departures. These gifts of time allowed workers to take a sick parent to the doctor or attend parent-teacher conferences for a child without incurring wage losses. Such gifts prevented workers from having to choose between paying the bills and caring for kin. Occasionally, older adults told me they would intentionally sign time sheets and tell workers to take the day off as a birthday or Christmas gift.[7] Workers reciprocated older adults' material assistance by providing flexible, empathic care—working extra hours without pay, doing tasks not authorized by agency care plans, engaging in relations that helped older adults' lives feel familiar. Taken together, workers' and older adults' practices of reciprocity embedded the official, bureaucratically supervised exchange of care labor for minimum wages within ethically complex interdependent relationships.

Agency policies frame gift exchanges as producing dangerous and exploitative entanglements between workers and older adults. Prohibitions against unmediated exchanges implicitly recognize the profound vulnerabilities of both home care workers and older adults. They are intended to protect clients from workers who might play upon the sympathies of a lonely old person to gain access to his or her accumulated resources or possessions. Agency policies thus frame older adults as vulnerable to exploitation primarily because of their dependence on others to maintain their daily lives. Agencies also prohibit gift exchanges because of an implicit awareness that older adults frequently have more stable incomes and more significant assets than those who care for them. Even Plusmore's clients, whose eligibility was based on their limited assets, often were more economically stable than their care workers, thanks to Social Security. Agency staff and training programs told workers that policies against gifts were in place to protect both workers and their clients. In practice, without any way to prove workers' innocence, clients' (and their kin's) accusations almost always led to workers being removed from cases, if not fired.

Home care agency policies that restrict worker-client relationships imagine older adults as vulnerable subjects, no longer capable of making autonomous decisions to participate in moral forms of exchange without risking exploitation. Through gift exchange prohibitions, home care agencies generate older adults and workers as independent entities best protected by regulating flows between them. Yet for many older adults, independence was not produced through boundaries that limited their engagements with others, but rather through their reciprocal contributions to interdependent relations. Thus, as much as they relied on home care workers for bodily and domestic care, they wanted to support their home care workers by listening to and helping with their problems. Many older adults felt the wages care workers were paid for their labor did not adequately reciprocate the embodied empathy they valued in care. Home care agencies do not typically tell their clients how much workers earn. They also specifically prohibit workers from discussing their wages with clients, as well as other personal information. Nevertheless, many older adults were aware that their home care workers were struggling to make ends meet. Knowing that their care workers could not support their families on their low wages left some older adults incensed. Many sought to restore a sense of balanced exchange through gift-giving. Thus, older adults proffered gifts small and large, many of which helped workers fill in the gaps between the money, time, and other resources needed by their families and those they received in compensation for their care work. Offering these gifts is one way that older adults see themselves acting as moral, equal, "independent" partners in interdependent social relationships.

In attempting to limit older adults' reciprocal exchanges with workers, agencies imagine older adults as vulnerable persons whose independence is threatened, meaning they require protection. Yet agency policies and the broader failures of capitalist markets to sustainably structure and remunerate care work generate these very vulnerabilities. These structures create the conditions in which workers are forced to choose between accepting an illicit gift or not being able to pay their bills.

"Too Much Going On"

If Doris's firing highlighted conflicts between agency policies and the interdependence of workers and older adults, the end of Grace's relationship with Margee and Belltower underscored the trouble agencies have accommodating workers' interdependence with their own kin. When Carmen first introduced me to Grace, she told me that Grace was an excellent home care worker. She was willing to take on the very hardest cases, worked tirelessly, and had mastered the ability of being simultaneously firm and gentle with clients. She also told me that Grace needed to focus on her responsibilities at work and let other family members deal with crises within her widespread kinship network. Grace periodically missed work to care for her granddaughter or take one of her parents to the hospital. Carmen thought Grace should insist that one of her five brothers and sisters help her parents instead. Grace later told me that her siblings usually looked after her mother, but had cut their father out of their lives because of his abusive past. She was proud that her siblings looked to her as the family's expert on caring for elders, though it meant some additional responsibility fell on her already overworked shoulders.

Grace normally arose at five o'clock in the morning, and looked forward to the days when her husband did not work. On those days, she could sleep in an extra hour because he could drive her to work. On a regular morning, Grace rushed out the door by 5:40 to catch the bus. Her husband walked with her to the bus stop a few blocks away, making sure nothing happened on the way. It took Grace three buses, each connected by a short walk, to get to the far western edge of the city where Margee Jefferson lived with her son Bertram. It was essential that each ride go smoothly and each transfer take no longer than its scheduled time, since any delays made Grace late for work, and Bertram left for his clerical job at a law office downtown by 8:00. Margee had a history of falling, so Carmen did not want the older woman left alone.

By 5:45 in the evening, Grace would begin preparing herself to leave the Jefferson house, knowing that she had only minutes to catch the express bus back across the west side to her north side connection. If Bertram was late, even by a few moments, she would be left standing and waiting for the regular bus, which might easily add another hour to her trip back to the south side. Several days a week, Grace would interrupt her cross-town commute to stop at the senior housing complex on the south side to visit her father, who was diabetic and had been blind for more than a decade. Grace had helped him access a variety of services, including a home care worker funded through the Community Care Program, and still stopped to visit him most weekdays in order to bring him cigarettes and prepare meals that he could later reheat in the microwave. After an hour visiting her father, Grace walked back to the bus stop to finish her journey home, spending a little time with her husband and granddaughter before she collapsed, exhausted.

Grace was able to maintain this backbreaking routine through the winter of 2007, when she lost her job with Belltower. According to Carmen, Grace had become too unreliable—she had missed too many days of work and failed to give adequate advance notice. Each absence left Carmen in a terrible situation, scrambling in the early morning hours to locate an available home care worker in time for the worker to arrive at Margee's home before 8 o'clock so that Bertram could leave for work on time.

Grace was fired because she chose care for herself and her kin one too many times. As far as I was aware, Grace had missed work three times on short notice in the previous six months. Throughout that time, she worked 50-hour weeks caring for Margee, trying to make sure the older woman's house still felt like her home while making it safe by thoroughly cleaning and reorganizing it. After Grace was fired, she was replaced by another worker, a quiet Filipina woman who was still learning English. When I visited Margee a few weeks after Grace was fired, the older woman was withdrawn and depressed, much as she had been before Grace came into her life.

Grace missed work with short notice after her grandmother died early one Monday morning in late September. When I visited Grace and Margee at the end of that week, Grace had returned to work, but not before being severely reprimanded by Carmen for missing work. As we sat and spoke in Margee's dining room while the older woman slept soundly in the next room, Grace was extremely upset, yelling and swearing (and then apologizing for yelling and swearing) as she told me what had happened.

Grace told me that less than an hour after her grandmother died, she called the Belltower office to tell Carmen the news, informing her that she would not be able to come in that day. Grace spent the previous night and early morning praying and grieving with her mother and sister. During the phone call, Carmen insisted that Grace had to go in to work. Margee could not be left alone. On another day, Carmen might have been able to temporarily substitute for Grace until she found another worker, but Carmen was alone in the office and could not leave. Grace recalled Carmen saying to her, "you've got other sisters, let them take care of your mother." This infuriated Grace. It was unthinkable that an employer would be so dismissive of her need to mourn with and care for her kin: "This is MY mom and it was MY grandmother who passed away, so I need to be there with my family."

After Carmen threatened to fire her, Grace tried to come into work despite her grief. She was at her mother's home in the distant suburbs, more than an hour away from Margee's house. Grace didn't drive, so she convinced one of her sisters to drive her into the city. On the way, her sister had some kind of anxiety or asthma attack. Grace had to call her brother to come and pick them all up, and they returned to her mother's house. She called Carmen again, explaining what had happened. According to Grace, Carmen "didn't care and said that I abandoned my client." Carmen told Grace not to come in to work the next day either, denying her the work and wages as a punishment for her unscheduled absence. On Wednesday morning when Grace returned to work, Carmen came to Margee's home and "yelled and yelled" at Grace, who remembered that Carmen "told me that I couldn't miss another day of work, that if I got sick I had to come in anyway." Worried about her job, Grace decided not to accompany the rest of her family to Mississippi to bury her grandmother next to her grandfather. She was heartbroken to miss the burial. As a child, she had spent every summer with her grandparents in Mississippi, "so I'm really used to spending time there and just so close to Grandma." She struggled to accept that her work caring for Margee prevented her from participating in this final act of care for her own beloved grandmother. Grace said Carmen also "wrote me up for abandoning my client," placing a written reprimand in her employment records.

Grace did not understand why her support and care for her own kin meant she had abandoned her client. It seemed reasonable to her that the agency should have a plan in place when workers missed work on short notice. Workers were only human, they got sick and had families of their own to care for. She did not see how it was her fault that Carmen and Belltower were unprepared for a predictable problem.

Carmen told Grace that the consequences would be particularly harsh if Carmen learned that Grace called in sick on a Monday during the two weeks Carmen would be on vacation the following month. This last warning infuriated Grace, who interpreted it as implying that Carmen thought Grace was lying about her grandmother to extend her weekend. Grace's tone suggested that she was deeply aware of the irony that Carmen would be on (presumably paid) vacation in a few weeks, but that she herself could not take an unpaid day to mourn or bury her grandmother without risking her job.

Grace next missed work without giving notice in late January, when her daughter was arrested in the middle of the night. Grace immediately took custody of her 18-month-old granddaughter, terrified that Child Protective Services would otherwise get involved. Her husband, who was disabled and diabetic, worked intermittently and had a job the next day. Grace told me that when she called Carmen early in the morning to say she could not come in to work that morning, Carmen told her that her granddaughter "isn't your problem." Grace was flummoxed by this response, saying, "Does she even have children? She wouldn't think to be so thoughtless about me needing to take care of Shani [her granddaughter] if she had kids. My daughter is young, and sometimes kids go through things when they're young. That's not Shani's fault. Shani still needs someone to take care of her even if my daughter fucked up. And there's no way I'm letting DCFS get their hands on Shani, because that will be bad for her whole life, and I ain't gonna let that happen." Grace refused to have the child cared for by someone she did not know, concerned that a child with limited language might not be able to report any abuse that occurred. Carmen refused to accept this as a valid reason for missing work on short notice, and wrote Grace up again, with the warning that another absence would lead to termination. Grace was exhausted and angry.

When Carmen came to reprimand Grace after this incident, she also inspected Margee's home. Grace distinctly recalled Carmen walking around the house, dragging her finger across all the furniture to see if it was dusty. Grace thought it was absurd that she be expected to keep Margee's house entirely dust-free, given how her client lived. "When I come in on a Monday after Bertram and Margee have been home all weekend and it's just disgusting. Bags and bags of garbage to take out of the kitchen, rotting food on the counters. This house is so disgusting it would be impossible to keep it clean, the dust is the least of the worries. I like a clean house, but it isn't possible to get this house that clean. Carmen coming in here dragging her fingers like that, really? And I'm not a housekeeper!" Grace found Carmen's detailed inspections insulting, in part because Grace kept her own home meticulously clean. Grace wished she could keep Margee's home equally spotless, but it was impossible given her client's lifestyle. Moreover, Grace insisted that her job consisted of far more than cleaning houses. It was her job to keep Margee healthy. This included her ongoing efforts to ward off Margee's depression.

Grace was unaccustomed to working for someone who was so unsympathetic and inflexible. She wanted to quit, but she couldn't afford to leave her job. Grace had spent years on the Chicago Housing Authority's (CHA) waiting list to move into a subsidized "rent-to- own" property. That year, she finally made it to the top of the list and qualified to move into a property. In the fall, she had found the perfect house for her and her family in a much safer and more convenient neighborhood. Grace had anxiously awaited the CHA inspections of the house. She was devastated when CHA had demanded the landlord make repairs to the building before her family could move in. By January, the house was nearly ready, and Grace started packing for the move. If she lost her job and her steady income, she feared she would be disqualified from the CHA program and would lose her dream house as well. Thus, no matter how poorly Carmen treated her, Grace was resolved to do everything in her power to keep her job.

A few weeks later, on a frigid February morning, Grace slipped on an icy sidewalk just a few feet from her home while running to catch her early morning bus. "I slipped and fell because it was so early in the morning and we didn't get a chance to shovel the snow on the porch. . . . We kind of heard the bus coming and I got kind of in a hurry and I was getting my bags and stuff ready to run and I lost my balance. Instead of falling forward, I fell backwards and hit my head on the stairs out there. I didn't know I had been unconscious for about 5 or 10 minutes or however long but I really didn't remember anything." She continued, "the only thing I knew is next my husband was standing over me and I was at the hospital. I had him call the job to let her [Carmen] know that I wouldn't make it in. He did that automatically anyway because I'm just like that. I don't like to call last minute like that. I like to at least call you 2, 3 hours ahead of time."

Though Grace was released from the hospital the next day, she had a concussion and sprained ankle. The doctor told her not to return to work for a week to allow time for both injuries to heal. When she called Carmen to tell her she was ready to return, Carmen told her that another care worker had been assigned to Margee's case. Carmen told Grace that she would have to come to the office to discuss her future with the company. Carmen hinted that Grace could continue working for Belltower if she willing to take a live-in case because such an arrangement would minimize the likelihood that Grace would miss work due to transportation problems or family conflicts. Grace was unwilling to take a live-in case, since she remained responsible for raising her granddaughter. Furious, Grace told me that she did not see the point of traveling nearly two hours each way to the Belltower office only for Carmen to harangue her.

As Grace told me about how she had lost her job caring for Margee, she tacked back and forth between describing the working conditions at Margee's home, her pride in having improved Margee's mood and living conditions, and her deep sense of injustice at how she lost her job. From Grace's perspective, Carmen took her job away from her because Grace needed time to care for her own body and her family. Grace was indignant that she could so easily be stripped of work in a home she had done so much to render habitable. She argued that the agency was still making significant amounts of money from her labor because now it was a safe place for another employee to work.

Grace, always an astute analyst of the conditions shaping her life, was profoundly aware of the ways that her caring labor had been exploited only to have her own needs disregarded when they threatened her employers' bottom line. "So I happened to get sick, and she's [Carmen] going to tell me that since I have a baby and I slipped and fell that I got took off the case. But I bust my ass on that case. I didn't make this your primary money case and then when I get hurt and I got sick days and time days up in there, you going to tell me that I got too much going on. Bull crap. I got a problem with that." She spoke breathlessly, her voice rising with her ire, "Now you want me to come in [to the office] and talk about it. What the fuck to talk about? I didn't bust my ass at this house for over six months keeping this house livable for you to put somebody else there. No, I'm not going to do full day live-in, I worked this case, I got to keep this case. This is the main case. I got a problem with that." Grace aimed much of her ire at Carmen's management. She believed that Carmen took Margee's case because of the substantial revenue it generated, but that it had been irresponsible to ask workers without the proper training or equipment to work in such hazardous conditions. Despite the inappropriate and unsafe circumstances, Grace worked hard to improve her client's home and life.

Despite her lack of specialized training, Grace did what she could to improve Margee's living conditions and her mood. She felt this was just the right thing to do. After taking a deep breath to regain her composure, she told me, "I just come in and do my job, you know. I was doing a very good job until I thought I had a little incident. She [Carmen] said I had too much going on. I had a sick path. But I had put a lot of time up in there so if I get hurt unfortunately, you're going to strip me from my case and tell me I got too much going on and abandoned my job? I had my husband call my job to let them know I slipped and fell and had a possible concussion. Now you want to send me somewhere else. I got a problem with that."

Notably, Grace did not argue that she deserved loyalty and consideration from her employer in return for working diligently, for low wages, in difficult conditions. Instead, Grace argued that her continued presence in Margee's home would sustain the improvements she had facilitated in the older woman's mood. Grace noted that Margee "would know when I got there. I could hear her turn over when she hears me coming through the door. Once she knew that I was there, she would just be happy." Grace predicted that Margee's mood would suffer in her absence, saying, "Now to take me out of there after I already got this lady back up, now you're going to shut this lady back down. What kind of social worker, what kind of person does this? You want to better the chances to make things better for in home senior care and then when you do a traumatic move like that, you are shutting this lady back down."[8]

Grace accurately predicted that the replacement worker would not be a fluent speaker of English, believing that Carmen employed immigrant workers who were less likely to argue with her. Grace deepened her moral critique of Carmen's actions by predicting that Margee's inability to communicate with her new care worker meant that the older woman would slip back into depression. "It took me forever just for her to get used to me. Now you're going to bring somebody else in there and now she's totally going to be lost. And to top it off, they don't speak English. How the hell you going to put somebody in somebody's house when they don't speak the same language? . . . How is they going to communicate? . . . Hell, you speaking whatever kind of language, there's no understanding there. Therefore, this lady [Margee] has no choice but to shut down. If she don't feel comfortable with you or she don't feel some sort of connection or some sort of genuine care, she's going to shut down." Grace argued that Belltower's economic interests were not in opposition to the moral and emotional commitments of workers, but supported by them. Even if Carmen's intention was to increase Belltower's revenue, her strategy of replacing Grace with another worker would backfire, saying, "When she [Margee] shuts down, you can kiss the baby's ass goodbye. You can kiss all your money goodbye because she's about to go on to la la land. When they get such emotionally like that and in her stage, she can't afford to get a shut-down like that because that will kill her. We are trying to keep her alive. We're not trying to get her dead and join her son and her husband. We're trying to help her. You can't do that to lift her up and then bring her back down like that."

Grace insisted that agencies needed to comprehensively consider the full range of care workers' contributions to avoid ongoing turnover of both clients and workers. Grace forcefully argued that good care demanded that agencies approach care as something more than a precise exchange of labor for wages, noting the many extra hours of unpaid care work she had provided to enable Margee to remain in her home. Care workers, in return, deserved a similar kind of flexibility and consideration for their own complex circumstances. She said, "You are going to lose a lot of clients like that and you're going to lose a lot of good workers like that when you don't give people a chance. Now, I've been busting my ass and proving myself for months. . . . And you work damn over a year and maybe have two, three, days taken off, come on." Grace contrasted the few days of work she missed with the dozens of hours worked without pay when Margee's son arrived home late. She said, "My hours was supposed to be from 8 to 6:10 and I don't leave out of there until 6:30 but I put on there [her time sheet] 6:00. And I'm not supposed to leave out there until the son walks in there. Sometimes he don't get there until 6:30 and I never once put 6:30 or 6:10 on that time sheet . . . Over a year's time, ask me how much time and money that I just gave away." Grace shrugged, "You want to tell me who cares and who don't care. It's not about the money, Baby. Sometimes you got to do stuff from your heart when you go into these people's places. I don't care if you're black, brown, blue, green. I don't give a fuck what color you is. If I see you in a predicament, I'm not going to let you wallow in it." Grace's forceful language echoed the moral exhortations used in home care worker trainings. Grace turned these moral arguments around, suggesting that unreciprocated gifts of time and money proved her dedication to care, while they showed that Belltower had unethically narrow economic motivations. Grace's critiques drew a direct link between care for kin and care for clients, suggesting that the agency could not exist without workers' moral commitments to kin. The least the agency could do in return was enable workers to care for kin without losing their jobs.

I met Grace at her home for the interview in which she made these critiques several weeks after she was fired. She was still living on the far south side, and I saw no evidence that she was preparing to move. Still unemployed, she told me that things with the CHA program had "gotten messy" and declined to elaborate. She and her family were struggling to get by while she fought for custody of her granddaughter. Grace noted that although her husband was often too ill to work and they were raising their granddaughter, the family got neither foster care subsidies nor disability payments from the government. She hoped that this might change when her granddaughter's custody was finalized, and she planned to return to work as soon as she could. She had little faith in the system. When I left her house that afternoon, Grace invited me to come back for a cooking lesson, as she had long promised to share some family recipes with me. When I called Grace a few weeks later to find a time to come visit, her cell phone was disconnected. I never heard from her again.

I next saw Carmen at a Belltower staff meeting. She told me that she had let Grace go because Grace turned out to be an unreliable worker. According to Carmen, Grace did not adequately prioritize her responsibilities to her job or to her clients. Each time Grace missed work, Carmen was left scrambling to find a replacement worker for Mrs. Jefferson. Finding substitute workers for Margee on short notice was particularly challenging. Many of the agency's workers were available to work half-day shifts on any given day, but substitutes for Mrs. Jefferson needed to arrive early in the morning and be available for the entire working day. As Grace intuited, Mrs. Jefferson's case was a lucrative one for the agency. Supervisors like Carmen faced ongoing pressure to expand their caseloads, ensuring ongoing employment for themselves and for home care workers, while ideally providing some revenue to the larger health non-profit of which the agency was a part. Belltower did not employ (and probably could not afford to employ) a bullpen of substitute workers available to provide substitute care on short notice.[9] This meant that whomever staffed Mrs. Jefferson's case needed to be highly dependable.

Carmen had not been able to find one worker available all five days. For the time being, two workers split the days, which Carmen acknowledged was not ideal given Mrs. Jefferson's personality.

Efforts to create independence out of interdependent relations obscure the ways in which older adults' well-being depends not only on the labor of home care workers, but also on workers' broader kinship and social networks. Carmen's explanation for why Grace lost her job—that she was unreliable, irresponsible, and had poor work habits—mirrored language widely used by the US media and poverty-reduction policies to explain why poor people have a difficult time finding and maintaining employment.[10] Carmen's description of Grace as having poor working habits also echoed "culture of poverty" arguments that rely on stereotypes of black Americans as lazy, irresponsible, and lacking in initiative to justify racial economic disparities.[11]

Describing home care workers (and especially Grace) as irresponsible or as having poor work habits insidiously misrepresents the causes of tardiness, absenteeism, and the unpredictability of their absences. Such explanations imagine low-income workers as completely autonomous individuals whose only legitimate responsibility is to their employment. However, as described in chapter 2, home care workers were often members of under-resourced kinship and social networks in which many members face periodic and severe crises. Home care workers sometimes have multiple family members with serious chronic illnesses, drug addictions, and/or persistent legal troubles. The home care workers I knew in Chicago were often one of few people in their social networks with income from formal employment. Home care workers were often treated as wellsprings of strength and stability by family members, and other members of their social networks often turned to home care workers for both material and emotional support.

For the most part, home care workers missed work because they saw no other choice—there was no one in their social network they trusted to watch their children or grandchildren, no one else who could successfully navigate hospital bureaucracies. Workers like Doris linked their own chronic illnesses to the ongoing strain of supporting so many people. They shouldered multiple stressful responsibilities and cared for multiple people. Without health insurance, when workers became ill, they were unable to rely upon formal medical care to speed their recovery. Unable to work, they lost valuable income, jeopardizing their ability to pay for housing, heat, electricity, telephones, and food. Too often one serious episode of missed work cascaded into multiple absences as workers struggled to keep themselves and their families safe and healthy.

Home care agencies, like most other low-wage employers, very rarely formally acknowledge workers' responsibilities to their extended kinship networks. Informally, many of the supervisors I worked with acknowledged that workers chose home care employment because it offered a relatively flexible schedule that allowed them to accommodate their families' child care and elder care needs. Belltower supervisors determined whether a worker's request for emergency time off was legitimate on a case-by-case basis. Most of the Belltower supervisors that I met were aware of the multiple responsibilities their workers shouldered, and worked to accommodate their needs. However, the lack of an official policy or wages for leave left workers vulnerable to the whims of individual supervisors. Carmen, for example, proved far less flexible than most supervisors in accommodating these situations. Without formal policies on family or sick leave, workers never knew how many absences would push their supervisors to terminate them and were often left pleading for flexibility and understanding. This contrasts sharply with the standard employment conditions in middle-class and professional jobs, where workers' family responsibilities are structurally acknowledged through the availability of paid sick and family leave.

Disrupting Interdependence

Capitalist enterprises like the home care industry imagine individual workers as discrete entities that can be understood, compensated, and penalized apart from the broader web of relations of which they are a part. Yet these relations are morally and socially present in every home care interaction. Lessons from mothers and grandmothers echo in home care worker's ears as they cook and clean. Anxieties about a sick parent or wayward child meld with anxieties about a client's depressed mood. Grace imagined Margee as her grandmother. Doris shared stories about her family with Mr. Thomas to fill the silence left in his wife's absence.

Many of the cases of turnover that I witnessed in Chicago resulted from the frictions produced by efforts to create independent persons by separating them from interdependent relations. The home care industry's endemic of high worker turnover has multiple direct causes. Sometimes these causes appear to be the fault of workers, such as borrowing money/theft, or missing work on short notice. Sometimes workers like Sally Middleton found they could no longer sustain physically taxing labor, as the accumulated exhaustion of caring for others for decades wore on their bodies. Nearly all the home care workers I knew hoped one day to leave home care work for better paying jobs in the health care sector. In most cases, the proximate cause of turnover was that workers could not sustain their care work amid the profound and ongoing social and economic insecurity their families faced. Their families' insecurity had multiple roots in the broader structures of racial and economic inequality shaping the American workforce, including the long-standing structures that push poor women of color into low-wage care jobs in the first place.

While current systems of care in the United States generate independence and inequality in tandem, generative labor can create other ways of living. High turnover rates and exploitation are not necessary to care for an aging population. The following pages discuss concrete changes in policy and practice to more fairly value generative labor and turn it toward the daily production of equitable interdependence. Such changes offer the potential to create sustainable lives at every age.

Conclusion

In the previous pages, I have argued that paid home care in the United States generates independent persons by capitalizing on inequality. In home care, two of the nation's most ignored and maligned populations—the old and the poor—are bound together by work meant to sustain both of their lives. Instead, the home care industry consumes its workers through policies and practices that conceive of older adults as independent persons whose well-being is separate from the well-being of their care providers. Conceiving of care as generative labor enables analysis that attends to the complex dynamics of care from multiple perspectives and across scales.

In developing the concept of generative labor, I build on the thinking of substantivist, intersectional, and black feminist authors to theorize both the antecedents and the effects of the mundane labor of making life in an economically, racially, and gender-stratified society. The concept of generative labor develops an intersectional life course approach to thinking about care that enables comparison across space and time. This conceptual framework understands the forms of moral imagination and habituated practice attached to Euro-American notions of care as historically and regionally specific. Within the framework of generative labor, any specific instance of care is analyzed by attending to the historical and personal experiences that generate the moral imagination and habitus of those involved, as well as to the specific bodily, social, and economic forms generated through this labor. The concept of generative labor thus connects past, present, and future moments of care; however, it does not presume that such labor is necessarily reproductive of previous forms of difference or inequality. Rather, the notion of generation leaves room for the ways that such labor makes life anew in ways different from, but still connected to, previous forms of living.

Americans take the labor required to generate life for granted, in part because dominant notions of liberal personhood require such erasures. Americans' reliance on care work (both paid and unpaid) is hidden both in interpersonal interactions and at the level of public policy. Nevertheless, generative labor—including housekeeping, child care, and other direct care for older and disabled adults, both paid and unpaid—is the work that makes all other work possible. Generative labor enables non-care workers to earn a living in other industries without threatening the lives of their families. Long the province of women who are expected to generate the lives of kin without pay, this labor remains undervalued even as it is commodified. Governments and corporations rely on families to sustain life, failing to recognize that the labor required is more extensive than kin can reasonably shoulder. These forms of moral imagination then shape contemporary arrangements and practices of care, forging concealed local and global webs of inter-reliant care.

Discussions of care often attend to the ways in which care relations harness affective and moral engagements or the ways that arrangements of care implicate inequality. I have shown how the moral and affective aspects of care are deeply entangled with social hierarchy and inequality. Social policies support the home care industry as a means to improve the lives of older adults. The well-being of its millions of workers is rarely centered in policy discussions or program evaluations. The profound generativity of care means that changing how we imagine, structure, and fund care has the potential to generate broader changes in how we organize social life. Creating a society that generates equitable lives for people of every age, ability, and social background demands fundamentally rethinking how we value and organize care. As I argue throughout this conclusion, this means rethinking the kinds of persons and social relations we seek to generate through care practice and policy.

Generating Persons and Inequality

Persons are generated as they are recognized by and participate in social relations. Therefore, different kinds of relationships create different kinds of persons. This approach understands personhood as changing over the life course as people's relationships and expectations for those relationships shift. In the United States, full personhood is extended to those considered physically, financially, cognitively, and domestically independent. Independence is a core American value understood as a necessary condition of autonomy and citizenship.

Public discourse rarely attends to the consequences of liberal personhood for our understandings of growing older, or to the risks of independence for those who are unable to hide their reliance on others. Many older adults feel that their need for care threatens their personhood by diminishing their social standing and leading people to treat them like children. Humans of every age are dependent upon others for survival, but in old age this interdependence becomes more visible. In the United States, independence is often generated by obscuring the myriad ways that poorly paid women—like home care workers—contribute to the lives of others.

To many Americans—including those involved with the country's home care industry—sustaining the continued independence of frail and disabled people seems like a commonsense way to imagine and pursue a good life in old age. This goal is inscribed in the authorizing legislation for many public care programs. Keeping older adults at home is assumed to sustain independence, while simultaneously ensuring that elders remain responsible for the costs of their food and shelter. Those directly involved in home care are less likely to see independence and cost-efficiency as obviously complementary goals.

Older adults in Chicago did not understand independence as a form of separation from others, but as a moral manner of being in relations with others. Living independently thus meant more than simply living in a private home rather than an institution. Older Chicagoans' understandings of independence were bound up with their broader moral imaginations. These understandings of how to live a good life among others were shaped by their very different lifetimes of experience. For older Chicagoans, independence meant being able to live in a manner that expressed subjectivities forged over their lifetimes. Eating familiar foods, visiting familiar places, keeping their homes organized in familiar ways. Being independent also meant continuing to participate in social relations in much the ways they always had. This meant hosting kin, sharing food, being supportive, and participating in meaningful conversations with others. For many older adults, remaining independent required them to form and honor social obligations, including those they felt to reciprocate the care that sustained their ways of life.

Older adults recognized that the empathic, personalized care that sustained their ways of life exceeded the mechanistic lists inscribed in agency care plans. While care workers' low wages might compensate for checking items off these lists, they could not compensate for the kind of empathically attuned care most older adults desired. To remain independent, many older Chicagoans felt compelled to reciprocate workers' care in other ways. Through myriad small gifts and favors, older adults worked to forge webs of interdependence with their home care workers. These connections made it possible for older adults to feel that they lived independent lives even as they grew increasingly reliant on others for daily assistance.

Care workers' dedication to caring in a deeply embodied and empathic manner is their gendered, raced, and classed inheritance. From family, workers learned the domestic skills they used in their daily work. These experiences imbued the mundane daily tasks that sustain households and lives with potent moral meanings. For workers, cooking was never simply about producing food, but also about sustaining persons, histories, and subjectivities. Cleaning homes was never simply about removing dirt, but also about creating familiar, comfortable domestic worlds. Home care workers learned to use their bodies as proxies for the bodies of their elderly clients. Drawing on this sensorial empathy, workers inhabited and reproduced clients' familiar ways of life. In the process, workers prioritized their clients' experience over their own bodily well-being, and simultaneously made their efforts less visible. In various ways, workers' race and gender helped to obscure their central role in sustaining older Chicagoans' lives. These forms of concealment protected their clients' sense of independence. By protecting clients from seeing the myriad and subtle ways that they depend on care workers, clients were also protected from feeling greater obligations to reciprocate.

Sustaining older adults' independence also meant disregarding care workers' embeddedness within under-resourced kin networks.[1] Workers began and continued working in home care largely because their families depended on their incomes, and workers initially felt that home care work would offer more flexible working conditions than other low-wage jobs. They were often frustrated to learn that the flexible working conditions in home care also meant that they often struggled to work full-time hours, and thus rarely qualified for the limited benefits and paid leave that were theoretically available at their agencies. Troubled public transportation systems and scheduling gaps between clients meant that workers were often away from their families for two or three hours beyond that for which they were paid.

Starved from the outside by inadequate funds and inadequate public will, home care depends upon workers even as it leaves them and their families vulnerable to ongoing economic distress and social instability. Neither home care workers nor older adults were deceived by these relations. Most were well aware of the value of workers' labor and the exploitative relations that organized care work. Workers continued to care despite these conditions because social policies demand that they must work to survive and support their families, even if that work generates perpetual precarity and bodily harm. Workers also insisted that their care work expressed their moral commitments and felt that they were a critical bulwark protecting older adults from the losses associated with aging in the United States. Workers found themselves cornered into providing care that far exceeded their job descriptions or any reasonable sense of what might be expected in return for poverty-level wages. Older adults' continued independence relied on these commitments. Care workers often felt like the last woman standing between their clients' continued ability to live in a manner that sustained their personhood and abandonment.

Home care agencies transform workers' moral values into economic value. Publicly funded agencies find their budgets constrained by low reimbursement rates, forcing them to provide care on very slim margins. Private agency budgets, on the other hand, are constrained because they must keep costs low enough for older adults to afford. Public programs rarely allocate additional funding to support worker training. Instead, agencies primarily rely upon workers' families to impart domestic knowledge to their daughters. Agencies extract these skills from their moral contexts, capitalizing on workers' experiences of kinship and care.

Home care agency policies and practices also generate workers and older adults as separate, independent persons by enforcing material and emotional boundaries between them. Agency staff hope that workers will develop the warm relationships with clients that make embodied care possible. At the same time, supervisors worry about workers becoming "too involved"—by which they mean emotionally, socially, and materially enmeshed—with clients. Supervisors use their own ethical discretion to determine when the limits of involvement have been breached. Concerns about workers and older adults becoming too entangled with one another reflect, but also regenerate, the understanding that such boundaries are necessary for sustaining independence. From this perspective, independence appears quite fragile, constantly under threat from predictable bonds that develop between people engaged in the daily labor of sustaining life.

These practices compound the structural conditions of home care. They threaten care workers' standing as independent persons by leaving them reliant on welfare benefits. Such practices also hinder workers' abilities to meet their obligations as members of mutually reliant webs of care. The social relations that sustain independence at the end of life simultaneously rely on, intensify, and obscure social inequality. It is not an accident of history that marginalized women disproportionately perform the moral and embodied care practices that sustain older adults' independence. Structural marginality makes care workers' contributions easier to conceal, helping their elderly clients appear independent. The policies and practices that conceal their contributions to social life make it increasingly difficult for them to be recognized as living valued lives.

Care in a Time of Growing Inequality

Inadequate public support for care weaponizes women's ethical commitments to care. One symptom of the invisibility of interdependence is that publicly funded care programs face perpetual attempts to slash budgets when state coffers run low. Despite its growth, the paid care sector is periodically threatened by attempts to shrink publicly funded social services. For example, the Great Recession of the late 2000s wrought economic havoc at every level, devastating household and government budgets alike. Older adults relying on retirement savings in the stock market faced profound insecurity, while deep cuts to state budgets threatened publicly funded care programs. Across the country, dwindling state revenues, induced by tax cuts as well as the recession, led to cuts in a wide variety of social safety net programs. Seen as expendable, home care programs proved particularly vulnerable to budget cuts.[2] Reducing public support for health and care programs may reduce taxes, but they cannot reduce the amount of care required to sustain meaningful lives. Despite cuts to public services and rising unemployment nationally, the home care workforce continued to grow, doubling in size between 2005 and 2015. Budget cuts and program shortfalls shift the ethical responsibilities for sustaining lives and social worlds to women in their capacities as kin and care workers. Underfunding care programs presumes that women (and especially those whose families cannot afford to hire paid care workers) will continue to feel ethically obliged to sustain the lives of kin and community members, bearing the bodily and economic costs of generating individual and social life.

The Great Recession accelerated trends that have been reshaping the US workforce for decades. People increasingly found themselves working in unguaranteed, part-time, and poorly paying jobs, and the available jobs are more frequently in health care and services. The future of work in the United States is no longer a future of producing things, but one in which most people work to generate life and ways of living. The economic recovery that followed the recession brought little relief to low-income families. Home care workers' wages, for example, fell slightly between 2005 and 2015, from $10.21 to $10.11 per hour (adjusted for inflation). The wage stagnation in home care jobs is one symptom of a US economy that has only grown more unequal. Home care workers' ability to access health care remains uneven and precarious. The Affordable Care Act (ACA), passed in 2010, expanded affordable health coverage to uninsured individuals. The ACA increased the percentage of home care workers with health insurance by 14 percent. However, more than a quarter of home care workers remained uninsured, many living in states that chose not to take advantage of the ACA's incentives to expand Medicaid eligibility.[3] Efforts to narrow Medicaid programs and eligibility threaten home care workers' health and their jobs.

In the midst of growing economic inequality, efforts to organize and advocate for domestic workers—including home care workers—have gained strength. These organizations raise the visibility of direct care work, arguing for the essential value of this labor.[4] In many states, including Illinois, the Service Employees International Union (SEIU) expanded organizing efforts and continued to bargain with the state to raise wages, improve training, and provide other benefits for workers providing CCP-funded services. The National Domestic Workers Alliance (NDWA), founded in 2007, successfully organizes domestic workers across occupational categories to lobby for legislation like the Domestic Workers' Bills of Rights, which extends state labor protections to domestic and home care workers. Home care worker organizations won significant policy changes in 2013, when the US Department of Labor extended minimum wage and overtime protections to home care workers by revising the companionship exemption to the FLSA. The regulations finally went into effect in 2016 after the defeat of lawsuits filed by the large home care corporations and professional associations.[5] Legal recognition of home care workers as employees entitled to the same protections as other US workers is a vital, but preliminary, step in recognizing care as essential economic and social labor.[6]

Whether or not the United States develops a caring economy, a large and growing care economy displaced the industrial economy that dominated the twentieth century. Industrial logics and work structures are a poor fit for the kinds of labor required in the care economy. And the neoliberal logics that arose in the late twentieth century—logics that prioritize private ownership and individual responsibility—are inadequate to face an aging population of overburdened and overstretched families. Moreover, nuclear families have never been able to sustain the full costs of generating life. How might contemporary countries develop care economies that facilitate equitable interdependence across families, communities, and generations?

Valuing Care

Broad policy reorientations are necessary to create an economy and society that facilitate equitable interdependence. This reorientation is necessary at every point of the care economy (child care, health care, care for people with disabilities, etc.). Scholars and activists have offered a variety of proposals for improving care work and creating a more caring society.[7] My suggestions here reflect and build upon these discussions. I focus on the ways that changes to care practice and policy can better attend to their potential for generating either desired or unsustainable forms of life. While these recommendations are tailored to the specificities of the home care industry, similar strategies might help other sectors of the care economy stabilize and thrive. Just as the challenges facing home care work arise at different scales of interaction, so too must efforts to build a society that better values the generativity of care work.

Though many efforts to improve home care work will focus on interventions with care workers, agencies, and public policy, changing the public discourse around care is an equally essential step. Organizations like the NDWA and the Caring Across Generations coalition have begun this work, raising awareness of the working conditions and importance of domestic and care work while advocating for concrete policy changes. Continued change depends also on older adults, families, social workers, care managers, medical professionals, and geriatricians re-examining basic assumptions about care work and old age. This means expanding conversations about what constitutes a good old age beyond the impossible and violent fictions of liberal personhood. It means an honest accounting of the histories, beliefs, and practices that turn the labor of generating life into a mechanism of racial, class, and gender exploitation. It means developing valued forms of sociality that recognize and reward the economic and social value of this labor. And it demands a profound reconsideration of what constitutes the good life that celebrates the ways that humans depend on one another to make ever-longer lives, together.

Compensating Care

Building a stable and skilled care workforce large enough to meet current and future demand will be impossible if care workers cannot rely on these jobs to provide the living wages and benefits necessary to sustain their lives and families. Historically, critics have charged that higher wages in caring professions might attract mercenary carers—individuals who perform care work just for the money rather than because of their ethical commitments to care. Such critiques of paid care are so widespread that home care workers sought to dispel them. Workers regularly told me that purely economic motives are antithetical to good care. For example, Grace said, "It's not about the money, Baby. Sometimes you got to do stuff from your heart when you go into these people's places." These statements did not mean that workers disavowed the need for better compensation. Recall that most workers seek care work jobs because of their ethical commitments to kin, which they extend to their clients.

Like most Americans, care workers seek work that will provide their families with material security and stability. They prefer care work to other forms of labor because they find such work morally and socially meaningful. Yet without compensation and working conditions that enable them to sustain their families, many workers are unable to continue in this line of work. Inadequate compensation is a primary reason that care workers leave these jobs. By this line of reasoning, improving compensation is likely to attract and retain ethical and skilled workers, not mercenary, uncaring ones.

Improving care workers' compensation requires policy makers and agencies to think comprehensively about how care work can provide a sustainable livelihood. Raising care workers' wages is one step that must be taken in coordination with changes to other policies that ensure that care generates sustainable lives and livelihoods for people on all sides of the care relation. Raising care workers' wages is thus a necessary but insufficient step. The majority of the care workforce relies on some form of means-tested public benefits such as disability benefits, health/Medicaid benefits, and food and housing assistance. Wage increases may mean that workers' families no longer qualify for such assistance, and any economic gains are spent paying for housing and health care rather than allowing workers to gain economic stability and security. Wage increases should thus be implemented alongside other changes aimed at stabilizing the lives of low-income care workers.

A broader group of policies aimed at creating sustainable livelihoods for care workers and other low-wage workers is necessary to grow the care workforce and to reverse increasing economic inequality in the United States. Among the most important of these is expanding access to health care and paid leave to all care (and other) workers. Large numbers of direct care workers do not have access to consistent, affordable health care. Yet these workers play an essential, if undervalued, role in the American health care system; their exclusion from it undermines the entire system. Home care workers use their bodies in subtle and complex ways to provide care, which deepens the embodied toll of ongoing poverty. Direct care workers' illnesses are likely to last longer and their injuries go untreated when they cannot afford health care. Without reliable access to affordable health care, home care workers are prevented from receiving the life-sustaining care they provide to others. Care workers must also have access to paid sick and family leave. Without such policies, care workers are forced to choose between taking an unpaid sick day or exposing vulnerable clients to their illness. This predicament can easily translate into choosing between paying rent and protecting the health of elderly clients. Many workers leave home care jobs for positions that will not force them to make ethically untenable choices.

Valuing Experience

Home care workers become expert in running the households of and caring for older adults whose backgrounds differ radically from their own. Their expertise is rarely acknowledged either in training or by other professionals. Valuing care means recognizing the immense effort required to develop the bodily and domestic aptitudes deployed by carers and incorporating this knowledge in training programs, career ladders, and health care teams.

Developing training programs that facilitate equitable interdependence means recognizing and rewarding carers with long histories of experience. Care workers' expertise is derived from the complex forms of bodily empathy they develop among kin and through years of paid labor. That so many workers develop these abilities without formal instruction reflects their families' socialization and their own aptitudes. This expertise enables them to reproduce their clients' diverse ways of life. At the same time, many new care workers require opportunities to develop the complex ethical, bodily, and relational skills required in these jobs. In the current era, people of all genders are less likely to learn domestic skills either at home or through schooling than in previous generations. Care worker training programs can no longer take it for granted that sizeable portions of the workforce will inherit these skills from kin. Investing in care worker training programs denaturalizes gendered and racialized assumptions that the ability to care well is innate to women, and instead recognizes the immense familial investments required to generate care workers.

Historically, processes that formalized other healing practices and forms of health care (e.g., midwifery) devalued women's knowledge and skills and ignored the kinds of ethics and skills people learn among kin in favor of standardized and rational methods. Efforts to professionalize direct care work would be better served by celebrating and rewarding knowledge passed among women through familial and informal channels. Current training programs typically impart technical and medicalized knowledge to home care workers. As the home care workforce grows, workers may need additional preparation for domestic skills like cooking, doing laundry, or cleaning. Equally important, however, is offering care workers ongoing opportunities to explore the moral, relational, and emotional complexities of home care work. Preparing workers for these aspects of care jobs means developing innovative active training modalities that go beyond the didactic methods common in care training. Experienced care workers might be enlisted to provide such training through apprenticeship and mentorship models that recognize their mastery and create career ladders. Longer term apprenticeships and ongoing mentorship may likewise help new workers navigate the complex moral and ethical dynamics of home care.

Care workers' experiences can contribute crucial knowledge to health care teams. Home care workers are not formally included in health care systems or consulted by medical practitioners. Their exclusion is one consequence of the broader devaluation of care work. Care workers develop deep and dynamic understandings of their clients' well-being. Their ongoing presence and embodied knowledge of clients enables them to detect when clients' health deteriorates prior to a crisis. Care workers are often also tasked with implementing medical advice and lifestyle changes, such as specific diets. Including care workers in multidisciplinary health care teams would create a direct link between elders' daily care and acute/specialized health care. Through such teams, home care workers could alert other health care providers to subtle changes in elders' emotional and physical well-being. As part of care teams, home care workers could collaborate with health professionals to realistically assess how to implement interventions in ways that specific older adults find acceptable. Including care workers in health teams is a crucial step toward recognizing and utilizing workers' embodied expertise. More broadly, developing systems that recognize, and make visible, the profound contributions care workers make to social life has the potential to shift how we value generative labor.

Valuing Interdependent Relations

Public and agency policies insist on treating care workers as independent persons. These policies penalize care workers' and clients' uses of reciprocity to forge forms of interdependence they deem ethical. Policy makers and family members justifiably worry about vulnerable older adults being coerced by workers upon whom they depend. Expecting workers and older adults to cease such relations is unrealistic. Care workers bear the risk of these exchanges; when they fail, workers are likely to be penalized or lose their jobs.

Formally accommodating reciprocity within capitalist labor markets and state-funded bureaucracies is challenging. Better compensating workers would reduce the underlying causes of the most worrisome gifts. Yet even such measures are unlikely to prevent reciprocities from arising given their critical role in social relations. Rethinking the role of reciprocity in home care could strengthen home care relationships and encourage more frank assessments of interdependence. Moreover, serious engagement with the complex reciprocities of material and emotional care that occur in these forms is one example of the many ways that older adults also provide care. Rather than penalizing reciprocity, the home care industry and related forms of paid care should develop methods of incorporating ethical debate into professional development. It is essential that employers and policy makers begin frank discussions that acknowledge the endurance of reciprocal relations in care as well as the potential for such exchanges to become exploitative. Increased attention in care worker training and new client orientations to the complexities of these relationships would begin to build a broader conversation and nuanced practice around the ethics of reciprocity in paid care.

Evaluating Care

Reframing care as generative of social life requires more comprehensive efforts to evaluate the costs, process, and outcomes of public care programs, like Medicare and Medicaid. Public policies that fund direct care for older and disabled adults, as well as young children, primarily fund care workers' wages and benefits. Across sectors, the care economy creates significant and growing numbers of jobs that provide livelihoods for millions of American families. These programs are evaluated primarily on the amount, quality, and costs of the services they provide. Evaluations often ignore the significant role these programs play as job creators, and thus fail to evaluate the amount or quality of employment they generate.

Refusing to consider the role care programs play in employment means that policy debates do not contend with the full consequences of attempts to reduce program costs. When neoliberal calls to cut costs are implemented, the unfunded costs of care are disproportionately borne by those who have for generations sustained the costs of caring for American families. Underfunding care such that care workers must rely on other public programs to sustain their families' lives may reduce the costs of one public program only to increase the costs of others. In addition, low wages mean workers have less money to spend and they thus contribute less to public coffers, leaving local business and institutions like schools perpetually underfunded. Comprehensive evaluation would provide a fuller account of the actual costs of care, and would enable debate about the amount of public resources necessary to provide care that sustains the lives of care recipients and workers. Evaluating the consequences of care programs beyond their direct effects on recipients is one way of more fully valuing the generativity of care.

Toward Equitable Interdependence

Care in its current form generates longer but ever more precarious and unequal lives. The mounting care worker shortage derives from a system that values neither old age nor the labor that sustains these longer lives. To date, methods of providing care within capitalist markets have relied on the marginality of women of color to conceal interdependence. Most arguments for improving the conditions of care work focus on the dire consequences otherwise facing America's aging population. Ongoing care worker shortages prove the unsustainability of a system that attempts to provide care for an aging population by exploiting low-income women of color. Efforts to improve the compensation and conditions of care work have the potential to develop a care workforce that is both sustainable and valued. Ongoing and future attempts to address these challenges must attend to the long-standing legacies by which care work generates multiple intersecting forms of inequality. Rather than expecting care practices to adapt to the demands of capitalist commodification, perhaps our economic systems should adapt to equitably accommodate the messy interdependence that sustains life. As we invest more resources and energy into extending human life spans, we can also create forms of care that generate equitable forms of interdependence.

ACKNOWLEDGMENTS

It is fitting that a book emphasizing the powerful generativity of human interdependence should acknowledge the scores of people who have cared for and influenced me through years of research and writing. Gratitude, even put down in ink, does not discharge such debts. All errors and shortcomings of the text are my responsibility alone.

Though this book is not centrally about my family, our experiences—like those of my audiences—inevitably shape how I have come to see and think about aging, care, and inequality. That my kin are nearly as relieved as am I to see this book published is a sign of how profoundly they have contributed to its creation. My parents, Ray and Lindy Buch, have supported me in every way possible, going far beyond the call of duty. In their different ways, my grandparents Maurice and Sally Broad, and Allen and Betsy Buch, taught me about growing older, and shared the profound gifts of intergenerational interdependence. My brother Dan Buch is my lifelong interlocutor—challenging, questioning, and encouraging my ideas. Karen Jurist, my sister(in-law), is our wise and pragmatic sounding board, her perspective simultaneously new and familiar. Tom and Robin Hill graciously accommodated my need to write during family visits, and shared their respective expertise in the philosophy of ethics and in elder care. Sharon Bishop and Sidney Richman are steadfastly thoughtful and supportive. Ken Hill has been the loving, supportive, and patient partner every scholar dreams of, sustaining me and valuing my work, generously accommodating the many ways it shapes our life together.

As I have carried this project with me across cities and years, friends across the country have provided emotional and material support. Though many influenced this project in other ways, each deserves thanks for the sheer feat of keeping me going. My profound gratitude to Bridget Guarasci, Kate Livo, Katherine Martineau, Leah Nico, Aviva Pearlman, and Jessica Robbins.

This book has followed me across four states and three institutions. At each, I have received generous support and accumulated debts. At the University of Michigan, Ruth Dunkle first suggested that my interests in inequality and labor might find fertile ground through their intersections with aging. The depth and breadth of Gillian Feeley-Harnik's knowledge are matched only by her generosity—her insistence that abstract social theory be grounded in the "imponderabilia" of everyday life is at the heart of my anthropology. Karen Staller mentored me closely—among her many gifts, Karen modeled the challenging art of engaging across the intellectual spectrum, from abstract theoretical debates to concrete policy analysis. Tom Fricke encouraged me to write more bravely. Laurie Marx played a critical role helping me navigate the bureaucratic wilds of a complex graduate program. Numerous others influenced the development of this project, including Fernando Coronil, Stuart Kirsch, Berit Ingersoll-Dayton, Marcia Inhorn, Bill Birdsall, Lorraine Gutierrez, Michael Reisch, and David Tucker.

At UCLA, Alessandro Duranti and Tamar Kremer-Sadlik created a generative and constructive intellectual community and provided feedback on early versions of these chapters. Carole Browner provided generous mentorship, honing both my arguments and my writing. Jessica Cattelino, Douglas Hollan, Linda Garro, Jason Throop, Sherrie Ortner, and Ted Benjamin offered their time, ideas, and feedback in ways that helped refined my ideas and arguments. I am grateful to my fellow SSIP postdocs, Iris Hui, Loan Le, Asia Leeds, Jade Lo, and Sarolta Lazcó, for their thoughtful comments and feedback. In LA, Vanessa Díaz and Kristin Yarris provided critical perspective and friendship. Leah Nico and David Hatch supported and cheered this book's progress at every stage; they, along with Dagny, Tavish, Chauncey, and Forrest Hatch helped make Los Angeles home. Leah walked with me down every important path, and regularly asked when she would get to read this. It is my great sadness that I did not finish it in her lifetime.

At the University of Iowa, my department and colleagues have created a warm and generative intellectual environment. My generous colleagues, Erica Prussing and Emily Wentzell, have offered support, guidance, and commiseration throughout. I am also grateful for the support and advice I've received from Mike Chibnik, James Enloe, Bob Franciscus, Meena Khandelwal, Ellen Lewin, Katina Lillios, and Sonya

Ryang along the way. Shari Knight and Beverly Poduska are reliably patient and kind while efficiently enabling the rest of our work. In Iowa, Ari Ariel, Anna Blaedel, Whitney Carino-Marek, Nick Carino-Marek, Heather Bingham, Mark Bingham, Brady G'Sell, Andy High, Mary High, Alexis Ihrig, Alexei Lalagos, Yasmine Ramadan, Aaron Seaman, Emily Wentzell, Adam Yack, and Marina Zaloznaya gracefully accepted my absences and absentmindedness while offering generous camaraderie.

Early versions of chapters were shared with the UCLA Mind, Medicine and Culture workshop, the UCLA Culture, Power, and Social Change workshop, the UCSD Seminar in Medical and Psychological Anthropology, and the UCSC Anthropology colloquium, where they found thoughtful and incisive audiences. I am additionally thankful for the feedback offered by discussants and other colleagues who provided commentary on papers that strengthened my arguments: Joelle Bahloul, Paul Brodwin, Janet Carsten, Jennifer Cole, Karen Hebert, Sharon Kaufman, Sarah Lamb, Jean Langford, Jessaca Leinaweaver, Julie Livingston, Steven Parish, and Danilyn Rutherford.

I am one of those demanding scholars who learns through discussion—it has been my great luck and privilege to share this work with multiple individuals and writing groups whose debate and comments have improved each piece of this writing. My first writing group, including Danna Agmon, Laura Brown, Bridget Guarasci, and Monica Patterson, patiently and incisively commented on early drafts. My deep gratitude to the members of the Care and the Lifecourse writing group: Laura Heinemann, Julia Kowalski, Jessica Robbins, Aaron Seaman, and Kristin Yarris. Our ongoing conversations about care, generation, gender, and inequality have immeasurably enriched this book. At each stumbling point and hurdle, their skillful problem-solving and encouragement enabled me to continue writing. Matthew Wolf-Meyer has pushed my thinking in new directions. Katherine Martineau's perceptive questions and careful feedback always enable me to see to the heart of the matter; she has propelled me and this book from its inception. Carol Stack shared her writerly and scholarly wisdom, gave detailed feedback on multiple chapters, and pushed me toward evocative but unfussy prose. I am profoundly grateful to all.

I am indebted to the anonymous reviewers at NYU Press, who carefully read previous versions of this manuscript and provided helpful suggestions for revisions. I'm also incredibly grateful to my excellent editor at NYU, Jennifer Hammer, to editorial assistant Amy Klopfenstein, and to the marketing and production teams at NYU, for their careful and timely work guiding this manuscript.

The research upon which this book is based was funded by the Hartford Doctoral Social Work Fellows program, NIA training grant T32-AG000117 and multiple departments and funds at the University of Michigan. I have also received support for research and writing as a Social Science in Practice Postdoctoral Fellow at UCLA and from the University of Iowa.

My deepest debts are to the many individuals and organizations in Chicago that allowed me into their workplaces, their homes, and their lives. These include home care workers, older adults, SEIU organizers and staff, home care agency staff, home care advocates, and myriad others. Though confidentiality prevents me from naming them individually, it was my honor to know and share time with each of them. The words I have written inevitably fail to convey the richness of their lives and experiences. They were astute analysts of their own lives; my hope is that this book shares some portion of their wisdom.

NOTES

1 Names of both individuals and institutions have been changed to protect the privacy of those who participated in my research. I emulate the forms of address used by participants as a way of signaling the subtle ways that relational practices index the hierarchies of age, race, class and gender that pattern home care relationships.

2 People who provide everyday care in the homes of older adults and people with disabilities are referred to by a wide variety of labels, including caregiver, home health aide, home care aide, personal care aide, home health worker, homemaker, and companion. I follow prominent advocacy and labor organizations in preferring the term "home care worker." The other terms are misleading for a variety of reasons. The term "caregiver" implies that care is inherently a kind of gift. The term "aide" implies that workers assist other senior professionals, but most home care workers labor alone. Home health care services fall under different policy, regulatory, and insurance regimes than home care. Home health care is typically covered by Medicare and private health insurance policies; home care is not. Home health services are typically used for a limited period of time following an acute health crisis, and involve some specialized medical tasks as well as assistance with activities of daily living. Unlike home care workers, home health workers are required to have Certified Nursing Assistant (CNA) training and qualification. Neither of the home care agencies described in this book required CNA degrees of employees, but both looked favorably upon applicants with CNA training and experience. The term "direct care worker" is frequently used to refer to all workers who provide the most basic care for older and disabled adults in a variety of settings, including nursing home aides, hospital orderlies and nursing assistants, home health care workers, and home care workers. The Bureau of Labor Statistics includes home care workers in the category of "personal care aides."

3 Both home care workers and older adults practice complex forms of empathy within their relationships. While empathy is always an "ongoing intersubjective process" requiring dialogue that unfolds over time (Hollan 2008, 476), the empathic forms developed between workers and older adults are deeply asymmetric. Jason Throop (2012, 408) argues that empathy is a "multimodal process that not only involves perception, intellection, affect, and imagination but also the bodily, sensory and tactile aspects of lived experience." Notably, older adults primarily

engage in empathic processes involving imagination, affect, and perception, while home care workers' empathic practices involve all of these as well as empathy's bodily, sensory, and tactile aspects. These empathic asymmetries undergird and intensify broader social and economic inequalities between workers and older adults. For further anthropological discussion of empathy and intersubjectivity, see Duranti (2010), Throop (2010, 2008), Throop and Hollan (2008), Hollan and Throop (2011), and Strauss (2008).

4 Care plans are formulated in a number of ways, depending on the agency, described in fuller detail in chapter 3.

5 Many states, including Illinois, now require minimum training for home care workers; this was not the case when I conducted my fieldwork.

6 Many of the older adults and workers I knew in Chicago spoke forms of English not commonly found in academic texts and other elite venues. These individuals were powerful narrators of their own life experiences; this is best represented by reproducing their language as closely as written text allows. In quotations, I have chosen to preserve the grammar and speech styles of speakers, removing only filler sounds like uh and um. Ellipses in this and other quotes indicate places where I've shortened the quotes for readability, to avoid repetitions, or to manage space limitations.

7 Mol, Moser, and Pols (2010b, 13). Care practices persistently raise questions that pertain to right behavior and the good life. People engaged with home care regularly describe their care as motivated by a desire to do good and be good people. In this sense, care may be a moral practice (a practice having to do with questions of the good) even when care practices have consequences that many would consider immoral (e.g., exacerbating inequality).

8 Bureau of Labor Statistics (2014).

9 Both the proportion and absolute number of older adults in the global population are rising rapidly: in the century ending in 2050, the proportion of people in the global population over age 50 is expected to rise from 8% to 21%. In real numbers, this represents a global increase from 202 million people over age 60 living in 1950 to a projected 2 billion people over 60 in 2050 (WHO 2015). In the United States, the numbers are similarly impressive: the proportion of the national population over the age of 65 is expected to grow from 14.1% (or 44.7 million people) in 2013 to 21.7% (or 82.3 million people) in 2040. The proportion of people in the United States over the age of 85 is projected to triple between 2013 and 2040, growing even faster than the number of people over 65 (Administration on Aging 2014). Rates of population aging reflect broader social inequalities and are uneven both globally and within the United States. Life spans are shortened by poor nutrition, harsh working conditions, living in dangerous environments, and lack of access to high-quality medical care. While often presented within catastrophist discourse of an aging crisis, I understand these statistics as describing demographic trends that are creating new social conditions.

10 Though actual wages have risen in the past 15 years, real wages when adjusted for inflation have fallen by approximately 4.2%. See PHI (2015) for wage data and further discussion of the consequences of the low wages and benefits earned by home care workers.

11 The federal poverty line is regularly critiqued for vastly underestimating the resources needed to sustain a household because it relies on outdated assumptions about the relative costs of rent, food, housing, heating, and other expenses. Current research suggests that families need an income of at least twice the federal poverty line just to afford basic expenses (PHI 2015).

12 See National Center for Children in Poverty (2015) for further discussion of the public benefits used by home care workers as a result of low wages.

13 Wage data from Bureau of Labor Statistics (2015).

14 Back of the Yards was once an epicenter for critiques of the violence of capitalism. The neighborhood's poverty, pollution, and squalor were immortalized in Upton Sinclair's *The Jungle* (1906). In the midst of the Great Depression, Back of the Yards gave rise to both the United Packinghouse Workers of America, which became a progressive leader in the union movement, and the Back of the Yards Neighborhood Council, a coalition of existing neighborhood and parish groups that became the model for Saul Alinsky's (1989) community organizing.

15 Hochschild (1983). See also Stacey (2011) for a longer discussion of the meanings and uses of emotional labor for home care workers.

16 See Edin (1995) for a discussion of these dynamics prior to welfare reform in 1996.

17 In this formulation, I draw upon Lisa Stevenson's conception of "care" as "the way someone comes to matter and the corresponding ethics of attending to the other who matters" (2014, 3).

18 Generative labor provides a framework that analytically links the kinds of personhood, difference, and political economy generated by, for example, colonial concerns about interracial intimacies in Indonesia (Stoler 2010) and by new forms of neoliberal morality and citizenship generated through elder care volunteerism in Italy (Muehlebach 2012).

19 In thinking of care as one example of the ways that people organize and navigate interdependencies, I build upon Julia Kowalski's (2016) critical insights regarding the ways that Jaipuri kinship ideologies of seva order interdependence.

20 Glenn (1992, 4).

21 The distinctions between reproductive and productive labor are ideological, rather than directly reflecting some fixed or natural division. Marx argued that "Every process of production is at the same time a process of reproduction" (1976, 711). How people understand which forms of labor are valued as productive or reproductive (or if these categories are socially relevant) varies across space and time. Indeed, these categories themselves were produced within the very capitalist logics they seek to represent and are partly a result of the extraction of some forms of labor.

22 These arguments find their roots in the writings of Marx (1976) and Engels (1978) but are more fully elaborated by socialist and substantivist feminist scholars including Glenn (1992), Yanagisako and Collier (1987), Yanagisako and Delaney (1995), Lamphere (1987), Sacks (1989).

23 See Glenn (1992).

24 Engels (1978).

25 For discussions of "dirty work," see Anderson (2006), Jerivs (2001), Twigg (2000).

26 See Glenn (2010) and Dill (1994, 1988b) for extensive historical discussions of the ways women of color have been coerced into caring labor in the United States. For important discussions of the evolving role of migration and globalization in structuring care work, domestic work, and other forms of generative labor globally, see Coe (2016a, 2016b), Constable (1997, 2014), Romero (2016), Hondagneu-Sotelo (2001), Parreñas (2001), and Degiuli (2016).

27 Glenn (1992, 3).

28 See Colen (1995, 78).

29 Inhorn (2003, 35). See also Rapp (2000), Roberts (1997).

30 See Glenn (1992, 2010) for discussions of reproductive labor beyond biological reproduction. See Ginsburg and Rapp (1995), Rapp (2000), Franklin and Ragone (1998), Browner and Sargent (2012), Roberts (1997), and Mullings and Wali (2001) for anthropological discussions of the ways stratified reproduction impacts the biological reproduction of human life, favoring the fertility and reproduction of some kinds of people over others.

31 Estes (2001), Minkler and Estes (1991).

32 The importance of productivity for sustaining personhood is evidenced by gerontologists' promotion of "Productive Aging" and "Successful Aging," which are labels that emphasize the benefits that accrue to older adults when they engage in activities deemed productive, like volunteering. For gerontological discussions of productive and successful aging, see Morrow-Howell, Hinterlong, and Sherraden (2001), Rowe and Kahn (1998). For anthropological and critical analyses of these ideas, see Lamb (2017) and Estes and Mahakian (2001).

33 Bear et al. (2015). The Gens collective builds from the intertwined uses of the prefix "gens" that signals the etymological linkages between concepts like gender, generation, and generativity and plays a crucial role in early anthropological theorizations of kinship (Bear et al. 2015; Feeley-Harnik 2002).

34 Thanks to Jessica Robbins for the useful phrasing distinguishing categories of practice from categories of analysis. Unlike the older anthropological parlance of "etic" and "emic," the language of categories of practice and analysis does not insist on an "insider" vs. "outsider" perspective. For an anthropologist working "at home," this distinction is helpful for considering the ways in which *care* as a category of practice that is deeply familiar to North American and European anthropologists has perhaps been too-seamlessly used as a category of analysis without interrogating its cultural baggage.

35 I follow anthropologist T. O. Beidelman, who understood imagination as primarily having to do with moral rather than epistemological problems. He argues that "what we know is embedded in what we believe, the latter being a base of assumptions and assertions from which we derive our decisions about what is possible and what is real" (1986, 34). Anthropologist Julie Livingston uses the term "moral imagination" to describe "the ways we envision possibilities for a morally better or worse world than the one in which we live" which are simultaneously necessary for empathy (2005, 19).

36 This draws on the thinking of Bourdieu (1977, 1984) and Csordas (1993).

37 See Felicity Aulino's (2016) discussion of bodily care in Thailand for an example of the ways that assumptions about the moral motivations for care may limit comparative analysis. This comparative problem is analogous to the problem David Schneider (1968, 1984) identified for kinship. Scholars since have proposed the category of "relatedness" as a term that draws attention to the diverse and processual ways that people come to understand one another as bound to one another (Carsten 2000; Franklin and McKinnon 2001). I suggest that care, like kinship, is deeply bound up with Euro-American ideologies that travel poorly in comparative analysis, and that generative labor might better hold together the practices, processes, and relations by which people work together to make life.

38 See Gal (2002), Collier and Yanagisako (1987), and Glenn (1985).

39 See Zelizer (2005), Folbre and Nelson (2000).

40 Scholars such as Joan Tronto (1994) and Arthur Kleinman (2008, 2009) discuss this distinction, with Tronto offering a typology of care based in part on the relationships between caring actions and caring emotions. Certainly, for many in the United States, care is understood as a powerful enactment of morality and solidarity. For example, Cheryl Mattingly (2014, 5) considers the ways in which African American parents caring for chronically ill children engage in "ongoing moral deliberations, evaluations, and experiments in how to live." Arthur Kleinman (2009, 293) describes care as "a defining moral practice" of "empathic imagination, responsibility, witnessing, and solidarity with those in great need." Notably, these discussions focus primarily on the moral engagements of family carers rather than paid carers.

41 In contrast to these assumptions, medical anthropologists focused on care show that carers employed by institutions and bureaucracies are profoundly concerned with morality (Mol, Moser, and Pols 2010a, 2010b; McLean 2007; Brodwin 2013).

42 See Zelizer (2005), Folbre (2012), and Folbre and Nelson (2000) for discussion of the ways that US ideologies about the moral relationships between love and money affect thinking about paid care. Home care workers deploy these ideologies when they argue that their work is motivated by moral rather than purely economic commitments. For example, anthropologist Maria de la Luz Ibarra (2010) shows how Mexicana elder care workers in California understand their work as motivated by spiritual salvation, a concern for social justice, and their

critiques of global inequality. Home care workers in Chicago made similar statements when I asked them how they recognized good care and good work, suggesting that workers recognize that in order for their critiques of their working conditions to be seen as legitimate, they must demonstrate that such critiques are morally (rather than economically) motivated.

43 Stevenson (2014).

44 Garcia (2010).

45 Ticktin (2011).

46 See Cole and Durham (2007).

47 See, for example, Ferguson (2013), Wool (2015).

48 Theories of personhood are described in greater detail in chapter 1.

49 See Iris (1988), Conklin and Morgan (1996), Lock (2003), Gawande (2014), Kaufman (2005).

50 Povinelli (2006, 5).

51 The association between liberal personhood and private property is embedded in Euro-American distinctions between the public and private spheres that animate capitalist democracies. See Radin (1982), Povinelli (2006).

52 The link between control over private property and legal personhood in the United States stretches back to the founding documents of the country, which guaranteed the right to vote only to owners of private property. Only property owners were thought to have the political independence necessary to vote without being influenced by the wealthier class (Hamilton 1775). See also Bachelard (1964), Radin (1982).

53 Radin (1982); see also Stern (2009).

54 Rowe and Kahn (1998, 42); see also Lamb (2014).

55 Attention to the forms of obligation that bind people in social relations and social worlds offers one way of thinking past the limiting logics of late liberal individual personhood. Elizabeth Povinelli suggests that social theory consider the relationship between obligation and power, noting that "being obligated to something does not mean you are determined by it. It is a much richer form of relationality, a continual nurturing, or caring for, bindings that are often initially very delicate spaces of connectivity. I think if one is open to the world—and by that I just mean being alive and having one's senses intact!—one will find oneself drawn to something, to a somewhere, to be bound to it . . . we then call this someone or thing or where to intensify this binding" (Povinelli and DiFrusca 2012, 84). Following this line of thinking, greater attention to generative labor can lead us to better appreciate, support, and build politics based on the forms of moral obligation and social power produced in care.

56 For discussions of personhood at the beginnings and ends of life, see Kaufman and Morgan (2005). For discussion of the relationship between different forms of generative labor and personhood at the beginning of life, see Carsten (1997), Conklin and Morgan (1996), Gottleib (2004). For discussions of care and dementia, see Taylor (2008), Cohen (1998). For discussions of care and personhood

among those diagnosed with brain death and persistent vegetative state, see Bird David and Israel (2010), Kaufman (2000), Lock (2003).

57 Supreme Court rulings, most significantly *Olmstead v. LC* (1999), upheld the rights of individuals with disabilities (including older adults) to receive care in home- and community-based settings, spurring a number of federal efforts to promote home- and community-based care.

58 Illinois Department on Aging (2016).

59 In actual practice, deinstitutionalization has led to community-dwelling people with significant disabilities receiving minimal public support or services and increased rates of homelessness and incarceration among vulnerable populations (Reaves and Musumeci 2015; Levinson 2010; Dear and Wolch 1987).

60 See Stern (2009) and Eiken et al. (2015) for further discussion of shifts in Medicaid funding for long-term care.

61 See Brodkin and Marston (2013) for extensive discussion, including international comparative analysis, of welfare-to-work programs, and see Lambert and Henly (2013) for a discussion of the mismatch between welfare work requirements and the contemporary labor market. See chapter 2 for a more in-depth discussion of welfare and welfare reform.

62 See Cronon (1991).

63 See Wilson (1996), Venkatesh (2002), Klotlowitz (1992). More recent work complicates these depictions by considering the role of informal labor (Venkatesh 2006), and of older and disabled adults (Ralph 2014) in Chicago's African American neighborhoods. See also Fennell (2015) for a nuanced discussion of the affective afterlife of Chicago's public housing projects.

64 See Black Jr. (2003), Grossman (1991), Hartfield (2004), Cronon (1991).

65 See Grossman (1991), Chicago Commission on Race Relations (1922), Cohler, Lieberman, and Welch (1977), Drake and Clayton (1993), Duneier (1992), Zorbaugh (1929), Hirsch (1998).

66 For in-depth discussions of global care chains, see Hochschild (2000), Sassen (2006), Yeates (2009, 2012, 2005). For ethnographic examinations of the effects of global care chains on particular families and communities, see Yarris (2017), Leinaweaver (2010), Parreñas (2001, 2005), Brijnath (2009), Colen (1990).

67 Heinemann (2013, 69).

68 Contemporary care chains primarily involve the migration of women of color from poor regions of the global South to wealthier nations, a legacy of the colonial practices of intimacy, kinship, race, and labor (Stoler 2010).

69 In the years since my fieldwork, Illinois became somewhat unusual when it stopped paying its contracts to CCP providers during a 2013 budget standoff, leaving agencies without the funds to pay home care workers for hours already worked. Though specific circumstances of this crisis relate to Illinois's specific political histories, it is common for home care to be one of the first programs cut when politicians seek to reduce budgets.

70 Mishel et al. (2012).

71 When older adults hire workers directly, they or their families technically become responsible for meeting all of the legal obligations of employers. Older adults increasingly rely on worker registry services (including new digital providers) that screen and match potential home care workers, but are not formal employers. For comparative and ethical purposes, my research focused only on older adults receiving services through agencies. In most of the country (except a few states including California), publicly funded services can only be accessed through agencies. Working within the agency structure provided a supervisory structure through which I received guidance and oversight. The agencies I worked with were chosen partly because they agreed that I would not be asked to report on individual workers or older adults. Instead, I provided each agency with summary reports describing general findings and topics of interest.

72 At the time of my research, the Illinois Department of Public Health was in the process of formulating licensing laws that applied to home care agencies. As of 2016, Illinois required home services workers to have eight hours of training at the beginning of employment, and eight more hours each year thereafter; registries and placement services are not required to provide ongoing supervision (State of Illinois, 2016).

73 The CCP is funded by a combination of federal Medicaid Waiver dollars, federal Older Americans Act funding, and Illinois state funds. In order to qualify for CCP services, adults must be age 60 or older, be a legal resident of Illinois and the United States, have non-exempt assets of less than $17,500, and have a significant level of unmet need. Because the CCP uses assets rather than income to calculate need, a number of low-income older adults do not qualify until they have spent down their assets. This means that boundaries between public and private home care populations are somewhat fluid. Many older adults learn about the CCP program during discharge planning after they have been hospitalized for an acute health crisis (Illinois Department on Aging, 2016).

74 All dollar figures given for wages and reimbursement rates are in 2008 dollars. In 2017 dollars, this translates to Plusmore earning a state reimbursement rate of $14.71 per hour of care and paying starting wages of $8.66 an hour. In 2017 dollars, Belltower clients paid approximately $21.50 per hour of care and paid starting wages of $7.64.

75 Belltower also provided live-in services to clients, charging between $180 and $200 ($203–$226 in 2017 dollars) per day. Live-in workers received between $90 ($101 in 2017) and $120 ($136 in 2017) for each day of work, as well as housing.

76 Belltower employees who worked full-time (over 32 hours) for three months qualified for health insurance benefits, six paid sick days, and seven paid holidays. Full-time employees were also eligible for one week of vacation per year, and those who worked more than six years were eligible for two weeks. "Regular part-time" employees, who worked between 20 and 31 hours, were eligible for six paid sick days after three months and seven paid holidays after one month of employment. Belltower's director was considering eliminating their health care

plan, since relatively few workers qualified, and even fewer could afford their share of the insurance premiums. Plusmore offered some limited paid time off on holidays: After 90 days of employment, workers who worked an average of 30 hours per week for the eight weeks prior to seven specified holidays were eligible for holiday pay on that day.

77 My observation of these meetings informs my overall thinking and analysis. I typically received permission to observe these events through meeting coordinators and group leaders. Due to the difficulty of procuring individual consent from meeting participants, I do not describe these events in detail. Boris and Klein (2012) provide an extended study of home care worker organizing in the United States, while Poo (2015) provides an extended discussion of the concerns and goals motivating the National Domestic Worker Alliance, which has been organizing home care workers since 2007. Meyer (2015) analyzes the critical role labor unions play for immigrant home care workers in Italy.

78 Supervisors at Belltower know their clients well and suggested older adults whom they felt would be interested in having someone like me visit them regularly. At Belltower, we contacted approximately 15 clients by phone. Four of the six clients who initially agreed to meet with me eventually enrolled in the study, as did all four of their workers. Supervisors at Plusmore have substantially larger caseloads, rarely meet their clients in person, and thus had less personal knowledge of their clients. Some supervisors steered me away from clients who lived in neighborhoods they believed would be unsafe for me to visit. We contacted approximately 60 clients by phone, I met with approximately 20, and finally enrolled 3 pairs in the study (3 more initially joined the project but dropped out after only a few visits due to illness). This selection method, though perhaps the best that could be managed considering the multiple recruitment constraints, had several obvious limitations. First, the simple fact that pairs were willing to share their lives and work with me for eight months suggests they felt they had little to hide. These older adults were generally proud of their homes and their lives, and the workers were generally proud of their work. Older adults who participated in this study were probably less wary of strangers and less guarded than the population as a whole. They may also have been lonelier than average. The exclusion of older adults with significant levels of cognitive impairment means that this study cannot account for the substantial challenges that dementia poses for home care workers and caring relations. Because I recruited workers through their agencies and clients, workers may have felt less freedom to decline to participate than clients did. To protect workers, I reminded them that their participation was voluntary at every point of the study and offered repeated opportunities to refuse my engagement. Over time, most of the workers grew comfortable enough with me to share personal stories, invite my assistance with their work, to visit them at their homes, and meet their families.

79 In such cases, I refrained from making such interventions, reminding participants that my confidentiality agreements applied to all involved.

CHAPTER 1. GENERATING INDEPENDENCE

1 In the United States, more adults live alone than ever before, an instantiation of ideals of independence (Klinenberg 2012).

2 Anthropologists such as Clark (1972) and Simic (1990) show that Americans have long understood older adults' reliance on children as demeaning and as placing an unfair burden on children. This contrasts sharply with places where the moral norm is intergenerational interdependence in which children reciprocate parental care early in life by caring for aging parents (Lamb 2000, Buch 2015a).

3 See Biehl, Good, and Kleinman (2007) for extended discussion of and ethnographic engagements with subjectivity.

4 For key discussions of personhood in anthropology, see Mauss (1979a), Strathern (1988), and Carrithers, Collins, and Lukes (1985). Lamb (2014, 2000) and Kaufman and Morgan (2005) offer critical discussions of the ways that personhood varies and comes to be at stake at different moments in the life course.

5 See Mauss (1979a), Taylor (1985), Povinelli (2002), and Ingold (2000).

6 See Salmond (2014), Dwyer (2017).

7 See Kirsch (2014), Shever (2010).

8 For examples of such denials, see Conklin and Morgan (1996), Gottlieb (2004), and Nicolaisen (1995).

9 See Kaufman (1986, 1994), Luborsky (1994), Lamb (2014).

10 For longer discussion of the linguistic practices that socialize US children into the behavioral norms of independent personhood, see Ochs and Schieffelin (1984).

11 The narratives presented in this chapter and the next are abbreviated from longer life history interviews I conducted with older Chicagoans and home care workers. Workers and elders had their own projects and purposes in narrating their lives as they did in these interviews. I expect that they would have spoken of their lives in different ways and revealed different aspects of their histories to other interviewers with other purposes. Workers and older adults could not help but be conscious that they were speaking to a young, white, graduate student who intended to incorporate their words into future publications for unknown audiences. I cannot know how they might have narrated their lives differently to people with different purposes or backgrounds more similar to theirs. I interpret our conversations and their narratives as necessarily shaped by the kinds of things they wanted me, and my audiences, to know about their lives. As is true with any personal narrative, the speaker's consideration of audience and concern for how their words would be understood does not make their words less true representations of their experiences. It does mean that these narratives are best interpreted as simultaneously historical, political, and moral speech. Weaving their narratives with my analysis I struggled—with inevitably imperfect results—to find a balance between offering my analyses and honoring their powerful perspectives. My efforts are guided by the work of narrative scholars including Garro and Mattingly (2000), Kleinman (1989), Behar (1993), Olson and Shopes (1991), and Hurston (2008 [1935]).

12 Theoretical discussions of personhood echo the growing emphasis on person-centered care in efforts to reform long-term care. Since the early 1990's, advocates of person-centered care have pushed for long term care reforms that prioritize care recipients rather than institutions and providers (Kontos 2005, 2006; McLean 2007; Basting 2006; Kitwood 1997). Some of these formulations have been critiqued by anthropologists such as Jessica Robbins (n.d.) as presuming a kind of "primordial" and universal person, existing outside of lived experience and social relations rather than historically contingent and located in social relations. One implication of my argument that understandings of personhood are dialogically produced within social relations and across the life course is that care reform cannot take the unit of the person for granted, and should attend to the ways that these understandings reflect and generate social hierarchies.

13 The Phyllis Wheatley home was part of a national network of organizations devoted to providing opportunities to African American women. It was established to provide "wholesome home surroundings for colored girls and women who are strangers in the city and to house them until they find safe and comfortable quarters." The South Side building accommodated 20 girls at the time (Chicago Commission on Race Relations 1922).

14 See Klinenberg (2001, 2003) for a discussion of the 1995 heat wave in which 700 deaths were attributed to the heat. The heat disproportionately killed older men living alone in single- room occupancy dwellings (SROs). In the intervening years, Chicago built a multifaceted system to identify and protect vulnerable older adults from heat-related death. Home care workers were asked to report any older adult living in overheated spaces, without air conditioning or adequate ventilation. In 2006, police, emergency, and other city workers were available to transport older adults to cooling centers. That August, 28 deaths were attributed to the heat.

15 See chapter 4 for further discussion of Sally's retirement, and chapter 6 for a longer discussion of the causes of high turnover rates in home care.

16 Ms. Murphy uses the terms describing social membership ("like a person") and biological species-kind ("like a human being") interchangeably. Like many Americans, Ms. Murphy employs biological understandings of species membership as central criteria in attributing social personhood.

17 Social death, in which individuals are excluded from the normal flows of social life, can hasten biological death through social neglect, withdrawals of care (medical and otherwise), and suicide (Klinenberg 2003; Scheper-Hughes 1993; Biehl 2005; Agamben 1998). Social death often accompanies physical exclusion or movements of people into marginalized "zones of abandonment" (Biehl 2005). In the United States, aging is associated with abandonment and social death when older adults move into institutional care; however, many community dwelling elders also experience social death (Klinenberg 2003). They fear social diminishment caused by losing their status as full adult persons, which happens when they are compared with, treated, and spoken to as children. Outside of the United

States, social exclusion is not necessarily a sign of the unmaking of personhood and social death but rather of powerful associations between older adults and spiritual worlds (Rasmussen 2012; Lamb 2000).

18 While girls and young women were often unable to avoid domestic work in Northern cities, they were better compensated and often able to find positions that did not require them to live in their employer's home (Chatelain 2015, 7).

CHAPTER 2. INHERITING CARE

1 Mullings (1997, 8).

2 See Solari (2006), Jones (2010 [1985]), Thompson (1963), Dill (1988a), Hondagneu-Sotelo (2001), Wang (2002).

3 Baca Zinn and Thornton Dill (1994, 5).

4 See Abel (2013, 2000).

5 For more detailed discussion of the treatment of older black adults under slavery and afterward, see Pollard (1981), White (1999). Available histories have relatively little to say about who provided care for free blacks without kin in the nineteenth and early twentieth centuries.

6 See Mullings (1997) for discussion of how persistent representations of black women as either hypersexualized temptress "Jezebels" or nurturing and obedient "Mammies" were simultaneously used to excuse sexual assault and to justify black women's consignment to slavery (and later domestic work).

7 See Glenn (1985, 1992) for detailed discussion of the racial and ethnic dimensions of domestic work in US history.

8 Though the term "the Great Migration" suggests a single migration, those traveling northward arrived in a series of waves. Approximately 1.5 million people traveled north between 1910 and 1930, slowed during the Great Depression, and then gained steam in the decades after World War II. See Boehm (2009), Black Jr. (2003), and Grossman (1991) for detailed discussion of the experiences of Chicagoans who took part in the Great Migration. Chatelain (2015) focuses on the experiences of black girls who migrated to Chicago. See Stack (1996) for narratives of Northern blacks who have returned to the South in recent decades.

9 Boris and Klein (2012).

10 Boris and Klein (2012, 22).

11 Boris and Klein (2012, 24).

12 New Deal compromises also excluded domestic workers from protections of the National Labor Review Board that regulates labor organizing and bargaining. Home care workers are able to organize when they are employed through larger agencies, but this has proven more difficult for those employed directly by older adults.

13 Fair Labor Standards Act (1974).

14 Many states implemented their own minimum wage and overtime protections, including Illinois.

15 Professional associations funded by large home care companies sued to challenge the Department of Labor's new rules.

16 The program is largely successful at keeping older adults out of poverty. In 2014, for instance, Social Security income raised more than 22 million people over the age of 65 out of poverty; see Center on Budget and Policy Priorities (2015).

17 Vladeck, Van de Water, and Eichner (2007).

18 See Roberts (1997). The Civil Rights and National Welfare Rights Organizations were instrumental in expanding welfare benefits to black families.

19 See Abramovitz (1989), Piven and Cloward (1993), Skocpol (1995).

20 For discussions of welfare reform and its aftermath, see Fraser (1994), Corcoran et al. (2000), Lichter and Jayakody (2002), and Newman (2001). TANF initially required recipients to begin working within two years of receiving benefits, and capped lifetime benefits at five years. PRWORA also authorized a number of "workfare" programs to help welfare leavers train for and find work. Evelyn Brodkin argues that workfare programs can thus be understood as "commodify-ing . . . valuing individuals based on their monetized contributions to the market economy, not their contributions to the family, community, society, or polity" (2013b, 7). Though PRWORA successfully slashed welfare rolls, in 2014, 22% of children were living in households with incomes below the federal poverty line, a proportion nearly identical to 1993 figures. Welfare-to-work programs funded through welfare reform help recipients find employment and provide tax benefits to their employers—many home care agencies participate in these. See Jiang, Ekono, and Skinner (2015), Parrott and Sherman (2007).

21 Romero (2016, 6).

22 Collins (1994, 50).

23 Chitlins are made from hog intestines, while headcheese is made from the animal's head, feet, and sometimes tongue. Both dishes are culinary links to pre-emancipation black households in which the only meat most slaves were given were parts of the animal owners deemed undesirable.

24 Doris saw her teacher's advice as supporting her dream to become a doctor. It is difficult not to read at least some amount of racial, gender, or class bias into this instructor's advice. Instead, she might have been directed toward other health care fields that require more training but also offer better wages, job stability, and opportunities for advancement.

25 Individuals receive Social Security disability benefits because they are determined to be unable to work due to a disability. In 2006, the average benefit was $938 per month (Social Security Administration 2006). People who are able to earn substantial incomes may not receive disability benefits. In 2006, the maximum monthly income an adult could earn and still receive benefits was $860. This creates strategies in which some people may try to work to supplement SSI payments without exceeding these ceilings (Social Security Administration 2006).

26 Equating older adults with babies and small children is common across the United States, where it indexes the marginal personhood of those deemed dependent. Anthropologist Aaron Seaman (2016) argues that spouses caring for partners with early onset Alzheimer's disease refer to their partners as being like their

child as a way of preserving kinship relations even when the marital relationship no longer feels appropriate. Similarly, Doris equates older adults to her daughter's children in order to emphasize the similarity in the forms of moral obligation generated through care.

27 During the 1980s and 1990s, widespread moral panics spread regarding sexual abuse of young children at daycare centers. While many of the cases that initiated this panic eventually proved false, they reflected widespread anxiety about the risks of large numbers of middle- and upper-class women entering the workforce during these decades. For women like Grace and Doris, whose mothers and grandmothers had worked, the threats of sexual violence were multiple and long-standing (Collins 2000).

28 See chapter 6 for a fuller discussion of this conflict.

29 Collins (2000, 200). See also Dill (1980).

30 Collins argues that black women's experiences in domestic work "fostered U.S. Black women's economic exploitation, yet it simultaneously created the conditions for distinctively Black and female forms of resistance." Collins argues that black domestic workers' intimate knowledge of white households and close relationships with white children led to a sense of "self-affirmation the women experienced at seeing racist ideology demystified" (2000, 13).

31 Dill (1988a, 36).

32 It is impossible to know how much of workers' presentations of themselves as morally committed to care are meant to defend against accusations that their care is immorally motivated by mercenary concerns. Workers had good reason to portray themselves to me as morally committed workers. Examples of women making claims to moral authority based on the importance of their work and the intimate cross-class/race knowledge they gain working in other's homes are widespread in the domestic worker literature. See for example, Dill (1988a), Colen (1989), Rollins (1997, 1985).

33 Across contexts, kinship and political economy are mutually constituted, and the forms of one shape the form and practice of the other, as evidenced by the importance of family ties in workplaces of all kinds (Smith Rolston 2014; Yanagisako 2002; Shever 2013; McKinnon and Cannell 2013). Modern attempts to purify capitalism of its constitutive kin relations serve the interest of capitalists by excluding the reproductive labor performed among kin from economic calculations (Glenn 1992; Engels 1978).

CHAPTER 3. MAKING CARE WORK

1 Mol, Moser, and Pols (2010a, 13).

2 See Graeber (2001) for extensive discussion of the relationship between economic and moral value. Lambek (2010, 2) describes ordinary ethics as "tacit, grounded in agreement rather than rule, in practice rather than knowledge or belief and happening without calling undue attention to itself." See Brodwin (2013) for further discussion of the everyday ethics practiced by frontline social service provid-

ers as they manage tensions between bureaucratic demands, state logics, and the needs of vulnerable clients.

3 Brodkin (2013a, 18).

4 Brodkin (2013a, 32).

5 Lipsky (1969, 1980).

6 These statistics also include frontline supervisors of personal care workers in related fields; data for elder home care supervisors alone are not available (Bureau of Labor Statistics 2015). Supervisors typically also earn health care and some additional benefits through their employers.

7 See Thompson (1967), Polanyi (1944).

8 Strathern (1996, 1988) argues that processes of cutting networks of relations are central to the generation of individual persons and related forms of private property ownership.

9 See chapter 6 for a longer discussion of these exchanges and their consequences.

10 See (State of Illinois, 1999) Section 815 for the full list of exempt assets.

11 Hull (2012, 259).

12 Frohmann argues that, in service sector firms, objectification is a primary function of documents because "defining the nature of its services is especially necessary for firms in industries delivering non-material products" (2008, 172–173).

13 See also Gupta (2012), Riles (2006).

14 Plusmore supervisors were typically trained on the job. The company's requirements for supervisors had changed over time. Long-time supervisors often had experience in health care, home care, or social services. More recently hired supervisors were required to have a bachelor's degree. It was not clear that supervisors received formal training or guidance in the ethical labor I describe here. Rather, supervisors discussed troublesome cases over lunch, across their cubicle walls, and sometimes during staff meetings.

15 Perm-temps typically were experienced workers whom supervisors trusted to have the breadth of skill necessary to adapt to a wide range of clients. They were guaranteed 40 hours of work per week, and thus a more consistent paycheck than regular workers. The position was considered a promotion for the most reliable and competent workers. This practice meant that no single client received the best care Plusmore had to offer, but allowed the agency to meet its service hour goals.

16 Frequently, instead of formally firing workers, supervisors refrained from offering them new clients. This saved them from the more elaborate, union-mediated process of terminating workers. It also created a reserve pool of workers available in emergencies.

17 QA supervisors were typically very experienced home care workers promoted to low-level management positions. QAs normally spent their time conducting CCP mandated biannual home visits to monitor workers' performance. They were sometimes called upon to act as supervisors' eyes and ears in the field, helping supervisors get a more complete understanding of a difficult client's needs and household. QAs and perm-temps also represented Plusmore's attempt to create a

(limited) career ladder for the best workers, increasing both their responsibilities and their wages.

18 Belltower supervisors argued that they needed to recruit clients to keep their workers employed, but they also hired new workers at a steady pace. When workers lost cases because a client died or moved to a nursing home, they often sought employment from a different agency if Belltower could not provide them with a new client that suited their schedule quickly enough.

19 See Angus et al. (2005) and Bourdieu (1984) for in-depth discussions of the ways that social differences manifest in aesthetic tastes and the embodied dimensions of daily life.

20 Typically used to describe linguistic behavior, the concept of code-switching describes the ways that individuals from non-dominant backgrounds are able to switch between dominant forms of speech and non-dominant forms depending on context. Home care workers display a similar kind of fluency not only in terms of speech but also in terms of dress, cooking, and bodily mannerisms.

21 In 2006, home care workers were not protected by federal minimum wage and overtime protections, but they were protected by Illinois state law.

22 I have chosen not to further specify the wife's country of origin, attempting to balance between protecting these clients' identities (their countries of origin render them easily recognizable at Belltower) and the importance of her heritage in the story at hand.

CHAPTER 4. EMBODYING INEQUALITY

1 See Csordas (1993) for greater discussion of the body as the experiential ground for culture, morality, and social life.

2 This process is not unique to old age, but rather appears common across the life course in contexts of care with individuals who are not easily able to efface their reliance on others. For example, Ochs and Schieffelin (2001) show how mothers efface their participation in children's activities through dinner table conversations, while Edgerton (1967) describes a similar process by which friends and family of people with intellectual disabilities efface the ways they help their relations survive in the community.

3 She spent two of these days with another Belltower client.

4 For lengthier discussion of the implications of these practices for theories of personhood, see Buch (2013).

5 Bourdieu (1984, 137).

6 Farquhar and Lock (2007, 2).

7 Mauss (1979b).

8 Geurts (2002) offers an extended case study of the ways in which people are socialized into different sensory and bodily capacities, and the ways that these capacities come to figure in moral evaluations and discourse.

9 See Tomori (2014) for extended discussion of American practices and ideologies surrounding infant sleep. See also Wolf-Meyer (2012) for a broad discussion of the

links between ideologies of sleep, bodily orders and disorders, and the demands capitalism makes on individual bodies.

10 Farquhar and Lock (2007).

11 Mol (2002).

12 Bourdieu (1977, 1984).

13 Mauss first used the term "habitus" to highlight the "acquired ability" aspects of body techniques. He argued that, unlike individual habits, habitus varies especially "between societies, educations, properties and fashions, prestiges. We should see them as the techniques and work of collective and individual practical reason rather than merely the soul and its repetitive faculties" (1979b, 53). Bourdieu popularized and elaborated the term, describing habitus as the outcome of practice, and the dispositions of habitus as a signficant engine of social difference and inequality.

14 Bourdieu (1984).

15 Haraway (1991, 10).

16 Mol (2008), Mol, Moser, and Pols (2010b).

17 Anthropologists working across the globe find that care work shapes subjectivity, morality, and political action in complex ways. For examples, see Danely (2016) and Ibarra (2002, 2010, 2003, 2013).

CHAPTER 5. INDEPENDENT LIVING

1 See Perry (2014b, 2014a), Leibing, Guberman, and Wiles (2016, 2011) for discussions of the ways that aging in place and concerns over institutionalization manifest in the United States, Canada, and New Zealand.

2 Carsten and Hugh-Jones (1995, 2–3).

3 Nursing homes are not inherently or necessarily sites of abandonment and social death, even if aging Chicagoans perceived them that way. Nursing homes are also liminal spaces (Shield 1990). Personhood and sociality may be sustained, recuperated, and transformed within nursing homes and other sites of institutional care (Chaterjee 2006; McLean 2007; Robbins 2013).

4 Lévi-Strauss (1987).

5 Bahloul (1996), Buch (2015b), Marcoux (2001).

6 See Heinemann (2016).

7 Block (2016, 157).

8 Fennell (2015).

9 Mrs. Silverman's comment reflects widespread assumptions among white employers of domestic workers about how workers prefer to be treated despite significant critiques of such assumptions in black discourse and literature. One well-known example is Mari Evans's (1970) poem "When in Rome."

CHAPTER 6. CARE FALLS APART

1 Estimates of turnover are notoriously difficult to measure. Statistics typically account for agency-level turnover (i.e., workers who are fired or quit), not the

additional number of workers who are reassigned to new cases within the same agency. Both numbers influence continuity and quality of care for older adults. Estimates also fail to account for workers who leave one agency but continue to work in home care either at another agency or directly employed by clients. Even the most conservative of these estimates points to an ongoing crisis in home care, since replacing lost workers is expensive for agencies, and instability can compromise the health and well-being of elders (PHI 2015; Dill and Cagle 2010).

2 See Mittal, Rosen, and Leana (2009), Morris (2009), Dill and Cagle (2010), (Ejaz et al. 2015).

3 At Belltower, unmediated gifts were prohibited, though supervisors told me they sometimes allowed clients to pay workers "tips" or "bonuses" funneled through the agency.

4 Zelizer (2005).

5 While scholars including Mauss (1990) and Bornstein (2012) show how gift exchange can be used to mitigate economic inequality, other anthropologists have shown that forms of reciprocal exchange play a critical role in generating the forms of difference that create the basis of inequality (Strathern 1988; Lévi-Strauss 1969; Rubin 1975; Graeber 2011).

6 See Buch (2014). For extended discussion of the links between gifts and gendered personhood, see Strathern (1988).

7 When Belltower clients signed time sheets for unworked hours, these were relatively straightforward gifts, since they paid for service by the hour. When Plusmore clients signed time sheets for unworked hours, the gift was more complex, including both a gift of the small co-pay that clients were charged per hour of care and the authorization for wages paid by public funds.

8 Grace's critiques have a great deal in common with the moral critiques made by Mexicana care workers in Santa Barbara studied by Ibarra (2013).

9 This was a notable difference between Plusmore and Belltower. Plusmore had a stable roster of perm-temps available to provide substitute care. With its much smaller size, Belltower could not afford such an arrangement, instead finding substitutes among its regular cadre of workers, few of whom had full-time work. Because of this arrangement, finding a substitute worker required time, making it difficult for Carmen to find a worker who could arrive at Margee's home by 8 a.m.

10 These perceptions are discussed in Edin and Lein (1997).

11 See Lewis (1969), and Office of Policy and Planning Research (1965). For critiques of the culture of poverty thesis, see Bonilla-Silva (2006), Bourgois (2001), Lamont and Small (2008).

CONCLUSION

1 Feminist scholars and activists have long critiqued the relative invisibility of care work and care workers (Poo 2015; Glenn 2010; Steinem 1987). The hidden quality care work is not incidental to the work of caring in the United States, but rather central to the practices that produce independent persons.

2 Attempts to shrink government spending periodically threaten home care services around the country. For example, in 2015 a budget standoff between Illinois's governor and legislature meant the state stopped reimbursing home care agencies (along with other social and health services providers) for services rendered; by April 2016, the state owed CCP providers more than $200 million. Smaller providers were forced to take out loans to pay their workers, as larger providers threatened lawsuits. By early 2016, major Chicago-area service providers were making drastic cuts to programs and services, leading to ever-longer waiting lists for publicly funded home care. For low-income workers in Chicago, cuts to social services were doubly devastating. These cuts meant job instability for those who provide services like home care and a reduction in the social safety net programs—like subsidized child care—that help workers support their families on low wages. These cuts coincided with a precipitous rise in violence in Chicago, which was disproportionately located in the poor neighborhoods where home care workers and CCP clients are most likely to live. See Fessenden and Park (2016), Sweeney and Corner (2016).

3 PHI (2016).

4 These organizations have developed innovative, intersectional feminist approaches to organizing, developing new strategies to organize those traditionally excluded from unions and working-class movements.

5 Contemporary efforts to organize home care workers, direct care workers, and domestic workers are rooted in longer histories of organizing among women of color. Nadasen (2016) shows that black domestic workers played a central role in the Civil Rights movement. They parlayed organizing skills learned in the Civil Rights era toward efforts to build a movement of domestic workers. The mainstream labor movement long ignored domestic work, focusing on occupations that (sometimes due to union rules) excluded African Americans and women. Boris and Klein (2012) provide an excellent history of efforts to organize home care workers in the United States. Though their history ends prior to the most recent efforts of the National Domestic Workers Alliance (NDWA), they foreground the necessity of radical intersectional feminist organizing to empower working-class women. It is precisely this form of organizing that Ai-Jen Poo and the NDWA practice (Poo 2015).

6 Whether the rule changes will significantly improve home care workers' incomes is unclear; in Illinois and other states, policy makers proposed prohibiting workers in publicly funded agencies from working overtime to avoid straining state budgets.

7 See, for example, Glenn (2010), Poo (2015), and PHI (2017).

BIBLIOGRAPHY

Fair Labor Standards Act. 29 U.S.C. § 213(a)(15).

1999. *Olmstead v. L.C.* US Supreme Court 527 U.S. 581.

Abel, Emily. 2013. *The Inevitable Hour: A History of Caring for Dying Patients in America.* Baltimore: Johns Hopkins University Press.

Abel, Emily K. 2000. *Hearts of Wisdom: American Women Caring for Kin, 1850–1940.* Cambridge, MA: Harvard University Press.

Abramovitz, Mimi. 1989. *Regulating the Lives of Women: Social Welfare Policy from Colonial Times to the Present.* Boston: South End Press.

Administration on Aging. 2014. A Profile of Older Americans: 2014. Washington, DC: US Department of Health and Human Services.

Agamben, Giorgio. 1998. *Homo Sacer.* Translated by Daniel Heller-Roazen. Stanford, CA: Stanford University Press.

Alinsky, Saul. 1989. *Reveille for Radicals.* New York: Vintage. Original edition, 1946.

Anderson, Bridget. 2006. "Doing the Dirty Work? The Global Politics of Domestic Labor." In *Global Dimensions of Gender and Carework*, edited by Mary K. Zimmerman, Jacquelyn S. Litt, and Christine E. Bose, 226–239. Palo Alto, CA: Stanford University Press.

Angus, Jan, Pia Kontos, Isabel Dyck, Patricia McKeever, and Blake Poland. 2005. "The Personal Significance of Home: Habitus and the Experience of Receiving Long-Term Home Care." *Sociology of Health & Illness* 27 (2):161–187.

Aulino, Felicity. 2016. "Rituals of Care for the Elderly in Northern Thailand: Merit, Morality and the Everyday of Long-Term Care." *American Ethnologist* 43 (1):91–102.

Baca Zinn, Maxine, and Bonnie Thornton Dill. 1994. *Women of Color in U.S. Society.* Philadelphia: Temple University Press.

Bachelard, Gaston. 1964. *The Poetics of Space.* New York: Orion Press.

Bahloul, Joelle. 1996. *The Architecture of Memory: A Jewish-Muslim Household in Colonial Algeria 1937–1962.* Cambridge: Cambridge University Press.

Basting, Anne Davis. 2006. "Creative Storytelling and Self-Expression Among People with Dementia." In *Thinking about Dementia: Culture, Loss, and the Anthropology of Senility*, edited by Annette Leibing and Lawrence Cohen, 180–194. New Brunswick, NJ: Rutgers University Press.

Bear, Laura, Karen Ho, Anna Tsing, and Sylvia Yanagisako. 2015. Gens: A Feminist Manifesto for the Study of Capitalism. *Cultural Anthropology Fieldsights.* www.cultanth.org.

Behar, Ruth. 1993. *Translated Woman: Crossing the Border with Esperanza's Story*. Boston: Beacon Press.

Beidelman, T. O. 1986. *Moral Imagination in Kaguru Modes of Thought*. Bloomington: Indiana University Press.

Biehl, João. 2005. *Vita: Life in a Zone of Social Abandonment*. Berkeley: University of California Press.

Biehl, João, Byron Good, and Arthur Kleinman, eds. 2007. *Subjectivity: Ethnographic Investigations*. Berkeley: University of California Press.

Bird-David, Nurit, and Tal Israel. 2010. "A Moment Dead, a Moment Alive: How a Situational Personhood Emerges in the Vegetative State in an Israeli Hospital Unit." *American Anthropologist* 112 (1): 54–65.

Black, Jr., Timuel D. 2003. *Bridges of Memory: Chicago's First Wave of Black Migration*. Evanston, IL: Northwestern University Press.

Block, Ellen. 2016. "The AIDS House: Orphan Care and the Changing Household in Lesotho." *Anthropology Quarterly* 89 (1):151–180.

Boehm, Lisa Krissoff. 2009. *Making a Way Out of No Way: African American Women and the Second Great Migration*. Jackson: University Press of Mississippi.

Bonilla-Silva, Eduardo. 2006. *Racism without Racists: Color-blind Racism and the Persistence of Racial Inequality in the United States*. Lanham, MD: Rowman & Littlefield.

Boris, Eileen, and Jennifer Klein. 2012. *Caring for America*. New York: Oxford University Press.

Bornstein, Erica. 2012. *Disquieting Gifts: Humanitarianism in New Delhi*: Palo Alto, CA: Stanford University Press.

Bourdieu, Pierre. 1977. *Outline of a Theory of Practice*. Cambridge: University of Cambridge.

Bourdieu, Pierre. 1984. *Distinction: A Social Critique of the Judgment of Taste*. Translated by Richard Nice. Cambridge, MA: Harvard University Press.

Bourgois, Phillip. 2001. "Culture of Poverty." In *International Encyclopedia of the Social & Behavioral Sciences*, edited by Neil Smelser and Paul Baltes, 11904–11907. Oxford: Pergamon.

Brijnath, Bianca. 2009. "Familial Bonds and Boarding Passes: Understanding Caregiving in a Transnational Context." *Identities: Global Studies in Culture and Power* 16 (1):83–101.

Brodkin, Evelyn Z. 2013a. "Street-Level Organizations and the Welfare State." In *Work and the Welfare State*, edited by Evelyn Z. Brodkin and Gregory Marston, 17–36. Washington, DC: Georgetown University Press.

Brodkin, Evelyn Z. 2013b. "Work and the Welfare State." In *Work and the Welfare State*, edited by Evelyn Z. Brodkin and Gregory Marston, 3–16. Washington, DC: Georgetown University Press.

Brodkin, Evelyn Z., and Gregory Marston, eds. 2013. *Work and the Welfare State*. Washington, DC: Georgetown University Press.

Brodwin, Paul 2013. *Everyday Ethics: Voices from the Front Line of Community Psychiatry*. Berkeley: University of California Press.

Browner, Carole, and Carolyn Sargent. 2012. *Reproduction, Globalization and the State: New Theoretical and Ethnographic Perspectives.* Durham, NC: Duke University Press.

Buch, Elana. 2013. "Senses of Care: Embodying Inequality and Sustaining Personhood in the Care of Older Adults in Chicago." *American Ethnologist* 40 (4):637–650.

Buch, Elana. 2014. "Troubling Gifts of Care: Vulnerable Persons and Threatening Exchanges in Chicago's Home Care Industry." *Medical Anthropology Quarterly* 28 (4):599–615.

Buch, Elana. 2015a. "Anthropology of Aging and Care." *Annual Review of Anthropology* 44:277–293.

Buch, Elana. 2015b. "Postponing Passages: Remaking Persons and Homes Through Paid Home Care in Chicago." *Ethos* 43 (1):40–58.

Bureau of Labor Statistics. 2014. "Occupational Outlook Handbook 2014–2015 Edition." US Department of Labor. www.bls.gov.

Bureau of Labor Statistics. 2015. "Occupational Employment Statistics." US Department of Labor. www.bls.gov.

Carrithers, Michael, Steven Collins, and Steven Lukes, eds. 1985. *The Category of the Person: Anthropology, Philosophy, History.* New York: Cambridge University Press.

Carsten, Janet. 1997. *The Heat of the Hearth: The Process of Kinship in a Malay Fishing Community.* Oxford: Oxford University Press.

Carsten, Janet. 2000. "Introduction: Cultures of Relatedness." In *Cultures of Relatedness: New Approaches to the Study of Kinship,* edited by Janet Carsten. Cambridge: Cambridge University Press.

Carsten, Janet, and Stephen Hugh-Jones. 1995. "Introduction." In *About the House: Levi-Strauss and Beyond,* edited by Janet Carsten and Stephen Hugh-Jones, 1–46. Cambridge: Cambridge University Press.

Center on Budget and Policy Priorities. 2015. "Policy Basics: Top Ten Facts about Social Security." www.cbpp.org.

Chatelain, Marcia. 2015. *South Side Girls: Growing Up in the Great Migration.* Durham, NC: Duke University Press.

Chaterjee, Roma. 2006. "Normality and Difference: Institutional Classifications and the Constitution of Subjectivity in a Dutch Nursing Home." In *Thinking About Dementia: Culture, Loss and the Anthropology of Senility,* edited by Annette Leibing and Lawrence Cohen, 218–239. Piscataway, NJ: Rutgers University Press.

Clark, Margaret. 1972. "Cultural Values and Dependency in Later Life." In *Aging and Modernization,* edited by D. O. Cowgill and L. D. Holmes, 263–274. New York: Appleton Century Crofts.

Coe, Cati. 2016a. "Longing for a House in Ghana: Ghanaians' Responses to the Dignity Threats of Elder Care Work in the United States." *Ethos* 44 (3):352–374.

Coe, Cati. 2016b. "Not a Nurse, Not Householp: The New Occupation of Elder Care in Urban Ghana." *Ghana Studies* 19:46–72.

Cohen, Lawrence. 1998. *No Aging in India: Alzheimer's, the Bad Family and Other Modern Things.* Berkeley: University of California Press.

Cohler, B., B. Lieberman, and L. Welch. 1977. Social Relations and Interpersonal Resources among Middle-aged and Older Irish, Italian and Polish-American Men and Women. Chicago: University of Chicago, Committee on Human Development.

Cole, Jennifer, and Deborah Lynn Durham. 2007. "Introduction: Age, Regeneration, and the Intimate Politics of Globalization." In *Generations and Globalization: Youth and Family in the New Economy*, edited by Jennifer Cole and Deborah Lynn Durham. Bloomington: Indiana University Press.

Colen, Shellee. 1989. "'Just a little respect': West Indian Domestic Workers in New York City." In *Muchachas No More: Household Workers in Latin America and the Caribbean*, edited by Elsa M. Chaney and Mary Garcia Castro. Philadelphia: Temple University Press.

Colen, Shellee. 1990. "'Housekeeping' for the Green Card: West Indian Household Workers, the State and Stratified Reproduction in New York." In *At Work in Homes: Household Workers in World Perspective*, edited by Roger Sanjek and Shellee Colen, 89–118. Washington, DC: American Ethnological Society.

Colen, Shellee. 1995. "'Like a Mother to Them': Stratified Reproduction and West Indian Childcare Workers and Employers in New York." In *Conceiving the New World Order: The Global Politics of Reproduction*, edited by Faye Ginsburg and Rayna Rapp, 78–102. Berkeley: University of California Press.

Collier, Jane F., and Sylvia Yanagisako. 1987. "Introduction." In *Gender and Kinship: Essays Toward a Unified Analysis*, edited by Jane F. Collier and Sylvia Yanagisako. Palo Alto, CA: Stanford University Press.

Collins, Patricia Hill. 1994. "Shifting the Center: Race, Class and Feminist Thinking about Motherhood." In *Mothering: Ideology, Experience, and Agency*, edited by Evelyn Nakano Glenn, Grace Chang, and Linda Rennie Forcey, 45–66. New York: Routledge.

Collins, Patricia Hill. 2000. *Black Feminist Thought*. New York: Routledge.

Conklin, B. A., and L. M. Morgan. 1996. "Babies, Bodies, and the Production of Personhood in North America and a Native Amazonian Society." *Ethos* 24:657.

Constable, Nicole. 1997. *Maid to Order in Hong Kong*. Ithaca, NY: Cornell University Press.

Constable, Nicole. 2014. *Born Out of Place: Migrant Mothers and the Politics of International Labor*. Berkeley: University of California Press.

Corcoran, Mary, Sandra Danzinger, Ariel Kalil, and Kristin Seefeldt. 2000. "How Welfare Reform Is Affecting Women's Work." *Annual Review of Sociology* 26:241–269.

Cronon, William. 1991. *Nature's Metropolis: Chicago and the Great West*. New York: W.W. Norton.

Csordas, Thomas. 1993. "Somatic Modes of Attention." *Cultural Anthropology* 8 (2):135–156.

Danely, Jason. 2016. "Affect, Infrastructure, and Vulnerability." *Medicine Anthropology Theory* 3 (2):198–222.

Dear, Michael J., and Jennifer R. Wolch. 1987. *Landscapes of Despair: From Deinstitutionalization to Homelessness*. Princeton, NJ: Princeton University Press.

Degiuli, Francesca. 2016. *Caring for a Living: Migrant Women, Aging Citizens, and Italian Families*. Oxford: Oxford University Press.

Dill, Bonnie Thornton. 1980. "The Means to Put My Children Through." In *The Black Woman*, edited by La Frances Rodgers-Rose, 107–123. Beverly Hills, CA: Sage.

Dill, Bonnie Thornton. 1988a. "'Making Your Job Good Yourself': Domestic Service and the Construction of Personal Dignity." In *Woman and the Politics of Empowerment*, edited by Ann Bookman and Sandra Morgan. Philadelphia: Temple University Press.

Dill, Bonnie Thornton. 1988b. "Our Mothers' Grief: Racial Ethnic Women and the Maintenance of Families." *Journal of Family History* 13 (4):415–431.

Dill, Bonnie Thornton. 1994. *Across the Boundaries of Race and Class: An Exploration of Work and Family Among Black Female Domestic Servants*. New York: Garland Publishing.

Dill, Janette S., and John Cagle. 2010. "Caregiving in a Patient's Place of Residence: Turnover of Direct Care Workers in Home Care and Hospice Agencies." *Journal of Aging and Health* 22 (6):713–733.

Drake, St. Clair, and Horace R. Clayton. 1993. *Black Metropolis: A Study of Negro Life in a Northern City*. Chicago: University of Chicago Press. Original edition, 1945.

Duneier, Mitchell. 1992. *Slim's Table: Race, Respectability and Masculinity*. Chicago: University of Chicago Press.

Duranti, Alessandro. 2010. "Husserl, Intersubjectivity and Anthropology." *Anthropological Theory* 10 (1–2):16–35.

Dwyer, Colin. 2017. A New Zealand River Now Has the Legal Rights of a Human. NPR broadcast. www.npr.org.

Edgerton, Robert B. 1967. *The Cloak of Competence*. Berkeley: University of California Press.

Edin, Kathryn J. 1995. "The Myths of Dependence and Self-Sufficiency: Women, Welfare, and Low-Wage Work." *Focus* 17 (2):1–9.

Edin, Kathryn, and Laura Lein. 1997. *Making Ends Meet: How Single Mothers Survive Welfare and Low-Wage Work*. New York: Russell Sage Foundation.

Eiken, Steve, Kate Sredl, Brian Burwell, and Paul Saucier. 2015. Medicaid Expenditures for Long-Term Services and Supports in FY 2013. Centers for Medicare & Medicaid Services.

Ejaz, Farida, Ashley Bukach, Nicole Dawson, Robert Gitter, and Katherine Judge. 2015. "Examining Direct Service Worker Turnover in Three Long-Term Care Industries in Ohio." *Journal of Aging & Social Policy* 27 (2):139–155.

Engels, Friedrich. 1978. "The Origin of the Family, Private Property and the State." In *The Marx-Engels Reader*, edited by Robert C. Tucker, 734–759. New York: W. W. Norton. Original edition, 1884.

Estes, Carroll L., ed. 2001. *Social Policy and Aging: A Critical Perspective*. Thousand Oaks, CA: Sage.

Estes, Carroll L., and Jane L. Mahakian. 2001. "The Political Economy of Productive Aging." In *Productive Aging: Concepts and Challenges*, edited by Nancy Morrow-

Howell, James Hinterlong, and Michael Sherraden, 197–213. Baltimore, MD: Johns Hopkins University Press.

Evans, Mari. 1970. "When in Rome." In *I Am a Black Woman*. New York: Marrow.

Farquhar, Judith, and Margaret Lock. 2007. "Introduction." In *Beyond the Body Proper: Reading the Anthropology of Material Life*, edited by Margaret Lock and Judith Farquhar. Durham, NC: Duke University Press.

Feeley-Harnik, Gillian. 2002. "The Ethnography of Creation: Lewis Henry Morgan and the American Beaver." In *Relative Values: Reconfiguring Kinship Studies*, edited by Sarah Franklin and Susan Mackinnon, 54–84. Durham, NC: Duke University Press.

Fennell, Catherine. 2015. *Last Project Standing: Civics and Sympathy in Post-Welfare Chicago*. Minneapolis: University of Minnesota Press.

Ferguson, James. 2013. "Declarations of Dependence: Labor, Personhood, and Welfare in Southern Africa." *Journal of the Royal Anthropological Institute* 19 (2):223–242.

Fessenden, Ford, and Haeyoun Park. 2016. "Chicago's Murder Problem." *New York Times*, May 27. www.nytimes.com.

Folbre, Nancy, ed. 2012. *For Love and Money: Care Provision in the United States*. New York: Russell Sage Foundation.

Folbre, Nancy, and Julie Nelson. 2000. "For Love or Money—Or Both?" *Journal of Economic Perspectives* 14 (4):123–140.

Franklin, Sarah, and Susan McKinnon. 2001. "Introduction to Relative Values Reconfiguring Kinship Studies." In *Relative Values: Reconfiguring Kinship Studies*, edited by Sarah Franklin and Susan McKinnon, 1–18. Durham, NC: Duke University Press.

Franklin, Sarah, and Helena Ragone, eds. 1998. *Reproducing Reproduction: Kinship, Power, and Technological Innovation*. Philadelphia: University of Pennsylvania Press.

Fraser, Nancy. 1994. "After the Family Wage: Gender Equity and the Welfare State." *Political Theory* 22 (4):591–6118.

Frohmann, Bernd. 2008. "Documentary Ethics, Ontology, and Politics." *Archival Science* 8:165–180.

Gal, Susan. 2002. "A Semiotics of the Public/Private Distinction." *Differences: A Journal of Feminist Cultural Studies* 13 (1):77–95.

Garcia, Angela. 2010. *The Pastoral Clinic: Addiction and Dispossession along the Rio Grande*. Berkeley: University of California Press.

Garro, Linda C., and Cheryl Mattingly. 2000. "Narrative as Construct and Construction." In *Narrative and the Cultural Construction of Illness and Healing*, edited by Cheryl Mattingly and Linda Garro, 1–49. Berkeley: University of California Press.

Gawande, Atul. 2014. *Being Mortal: Medicine and What Matters in the End*. New York: Metropolitan Books.

Geurts, Katherine Lynne. 2002. *Culture and the Senses: Bodily Ways of Knowing in an African Community*. Berkeley: University of California Press.

Ginsburg, Faye, and Rayna Rapp. 1995. "Introduction." In *Conceiving the New World Order*, edited by Faye Ginsburg and Rayna Rapp, 1–17. Berkeley: University of California Press.

Glenn, Evelyn Nakano. 1985. "Racial Ethnic Women's Labor: The Intersection of Race, Gender and Class Oppression." *Review of Radical Political Economics* 17:86–108.

Glenn, Evelyn Nakano. 1992. "From Servitude to Service Work: Historical Continuities in the Racial Division of Paid Reproductive Labor." *Signs* 18:1–43.

Glenn, Evelyn Nakano. 2010. *Forced to Care: Coercion and Caregiving in America.* Cambridge, MA: Harvard University Press.

Gottlieb, Alma. 2004. *The Afterlife Is Where We Come From: The Culture of Infancy in West Africa.* Chicago: University of Chicago Press.

Graeber, David. 2001. *Towards an Anthropological Theory of Value: The False Coin of Our Own Dreams.* New York: Palgrave.

Graeber, David. 2011. *Debt: The First 5,000 Years.* New York: Melville House.

Grossman, James R. 1991. *Land of Home: Chicago, Black Southerners and the Great Migration.* Chicago: University of Chicago Press.

Gupta, Akhil. 2012. *Red Tape: Bureaucracy, Structural Violence and Poverty in India.* Durham, NC: Duke University Press.

Hamilton, Alexander. 1775. The Farmer Refuted. *Founders Online.* www.founders. archive.gov.

Haraway, Donna. 1991. *Simians, Cyborgs and Women.* New York: Routledge.

Hartfield, Ronne. 2004. *Another Way Home: The Tangled Roots of Race in One Chicago Family.* Chicago: University of Chicago Press.

Heinemann, Laura. 2016. *Transplanting Care: Shifting Commitments in Health and Care in the United States.* New Brunswick, NJ: Rutgers University Press.

Heinemann, Laura. 2013. "For the Sake of Others: Reciprocal Webs of Obligation and the Pursuit of Transplantation as a Caring Act." *Medical Anthropology Quarterly* 28 (1):66–84.

Hirsch, Arnold R. 1998. *Making the Second Ghetto: Race and Housing in Chicago 1940– 1960.* Chicago: University of Chicago Press.

Hochschild, Arlie Russell. 1983. *The Managed Heart: Commercialization of Human Feeling.* Berkeley: University of California Press.

Hochschild, Arlie Russell. 2000. "The Nanny Chain." *American Prospect* 11 (4):32–36.

Hollan, Douglas. 2008. "Being There: On the Imaginative Aspects of Understanding Others and Being Understood." *Ethos* 36 (4):475–489.

Hollan, Douglas, and C. Jason Throop, eds. 2011. *The Anthropology of Empathy.* New York: Berghahn Books.

Hondagneu-Sotelo, Pierrette. 2001. *Domestica: Immigrant Workers Cleaning and Caring in the Shadows of Affluence.* Berkeley: University of California Press.

Hull, Matthew. 2012. "Documents and Bureaucracy." *Annual Review of Anthropology* 41:251–267.

Hurston, Zora Neale. 2008 [1935]. *Mules and Men.* New York: HarperCollins.

Ibarra, Maria de la Luz. 2002. "Transnational Identity Formation and Mexican Immigrant Women's Ethics of Elder Care." *Anthropology of Work Review* 23 (3–4):16–20.

Ibarra, Maria de la Luz. 2003. "The Tender Trap: Mexican Immigrant Women and the Ethics of Elder Care Work." *Aztlán: A Journal of Chicano Studies* 28:87–114.

Ibarra, Maria de la Luz. 2010. "My Reward Is Not Money: Deep Alliances, Spirituality, and End of Life Care." In *Intimate Labors*, edited by Eileen Boris and Rhacel Parreñas. Palo Alto, CA: Stanford University Press.

Ibarra, Maria de la Luz. 2013. "Frontline Activists: Mexicana Care Workers, Subjectivity, and the Defense of the Elderly." *Medical Anthropology Quarterly* 27 (3):434–452.

Illinois Department on Aging. 2016. "Community Care Program." www.illinois.gov.

Ingold, Tim. 2000. *The Perception of the Environment: Essays in Livelihood, Dwelling and Skill*. London: Routledge.

Inhorn, Marcia. 2003. *Local Babies, Global Science: Gender, Religion and In Vitro Fertilization in Egypt*. New York: Routledge.

Iris, Madelyn Anne. 1988. "Guardianship and the Elderly: A Multi-Perspective View of the Decisionmaking Process." *The Gerontologist* 28 (Suppl):29–45.

Jervis, Lori L. 2001. "The Pollution of Incontinence and the Dirty Work of Caregiving in a U.S. Nursing Home." *Medical Anthropology Quarterly* 15 (1):84–99.

Jiang, Yang, Mercedes Ekono, and Curtis Skinner. 2015. Basic Facts About Low-Income Children: Children Under 18 Years, 2013. New York: National Center for Children in Poverty, Mailman School of Public Health, Columbia University.

Jones, Jacqueline. 2010 [1985]. *Labor of Love, Labor of Sorrow*. New York: Basic Books.

Kaufman, Sharon. 1986. *The Ageless Self: Sources of Meaning in Late Life*. Madison: University of Wisconsin Press.

Kaufman, Sharon. 1994. "The Social Construction of Frailty: An Anthropological Perspective." *Journal of Aging Studies* 8 (1):45–58.

Kaufman, Sharon. 2000. "In the Shadow of 'Death with Dignity': Medicine and Cultural Quandaries of the Vegatitive State." *American Anthropologist* 102 (1):69–83.

Kaufman, Sharon. 2005. *And a Time to Die: How American Hospitals Shape the End of Life*. Chicago: University of Chicago Press.

Kaufman, Sharon, and Lynn M. Morgan. 2005. "The Anthropology of the Beginnings and Ends of Life." *Annual Review of Anthropology* 34:317–341.

Kirsch, Stuart. 2014. "Imagining Corporate Personhood." *PoLAR: Political and Legal Anthropology Review* 37 (2):207–217.

Kitwood, Tom. 1997. *Dementia Reconsidered: The Person Comes First*. Buckingham, UK: Open University Press.

Kleinman, Arthur. 1989. *The Illness Narratives: Suffering, Healing and the Human Condition*. New York: Basic Books.

Kleinman, Arthur. 2008. "Catastrophe and Caregiving: The Failure of Medicine as an Art." *Lancet* 371 (9606):22.

Kleinman, Arthur. 2009. "Caregiving: The Odyssey of Becoming More Human." *Lancet* 373 (9660):292–294.

Klinenberg, E. 2001. "Bodies that Don't Matter: Death and Dereliction in Chicago." *Body and Society* 7:121.

Klinenberg, Eric. 2003. *Heat Wave*. Chicago: University of Chicago Press.

Klinenberg, Eric. 2012. *Going Solo: The Extraordinary Rise and Surprising Appeal of Living Alone*. New York: Penguin.

Klotlowitz, Alex. 1992. *There Are No Children Here*. New York: Doubleday.

Kontos, Pia. 2005. "Embodied Selfhood in Alzheimer's Disease: Rethinking Person-Centered Care." *Dementia* 11 (4):553–570.

Kontos, Pia. 2006. "Embodied Selfhood: An Ethnographic Exploration of Alzheimer's Disease." In *Thinking about Dementia: Culture, Loss and the Anthropology of Senility*, edited by Annette Leibing and Lawrence Cohen, 195–217. New Brunswick, NJ: Rutgers University Press.

Kowalski, Julia. 2016. "Ordering Dependence: Care, Disorder and Kinship Ideology in North Indian Antiviolence Counseling." *American Ethnologist* 43 (1):63–75.

Lamb, Sarah. 2000. *White Saris and Sweet Mangoes: Aging, Gender and Body in North India*. Berkeley: University of California Press.

Lamb, Sarah. 2014. "Permanent Personhood or Meaningful Decline? Toward a Critical Anthropology of Successful Aging." *Journal of Aging Studies* 29:41–52.

Lamb, Sarah, ed. 2017. *Successful Aging as a Contemporary Obsession*. New Brunswick, NJ: Rutgers University Press.

Lambek, Michael. 2010. "Introduction." In *Ordinary Ethics: Anthropology, Language and Action*, edited by Micael Lambek. New York: Fordham University Press.

Lambert, Susan, and Julia Henly. 2013. "Double Jeopardy: The Misfit between Welfare-to-Work Requirements and Job Realities." In *Work and the Welfare State*, edited by Evelyn Z. Brodkin and Gregory Marston. Washington, DC: Georgetown University Press.

Lamont, Michele, and Mario Small. 2008. "How Culture Matters in the Understanding of Poverty." In *The Colors of Poverty: Why Racial and Ethnic Disparities Exist*, edited by Ann Linn and David Harris, 76–102. New York: Russell Sage Foundation.

Lamphere, Louise. 1987. *From Working Mothers to Working Daughters*. Ithaca, NY: Cornell University Press.

Leibing, Annette, Nancy Guberman, and Janine Wiles. 2016. "Liminal Homes: Older People, Loss of Capacities, and the Present Future of Living Spaces." *Journal of Aging Studies* 37:10–19.

Leinaweaver, Jessaca. 2010. "Outsourcing Care: How Peruvian Migrants Meet Transnational Family Obligations." *Latin American Perspectives* 37 (5):67–87.

Lévi-Strauss, Claude. 1969. *The Elementary Structures of Kinship*. Translated by James Harle Bell. Boston: Beacon Press.

Lévi-Strauss, Claude. 1987. *Anthropology and Myth: Lectures, 1951–1982*. Oxford: Oxford University Press.

Levinson, Jack. 2010. *Making Life Work: Freedom and Disability in a Community Group Home*. Minneapolis: University of Minnesota Press.

Lewis, Oscar. 1969. "Culture of Poverty." In *On Understanding Poverty: Perspectives from the Social Sciences*, edited by Daniel P. Moynihan, 187–220. New York: Basic Books.

Lichter, Daniel, and Rukamalie Jayakody. 2002. "Welfare Reform: How Do We Measure Success." *Annual Review of Sociology* 28:117–141.

Lipsky, Michael. 1969. Toward a Theory of Street-Level Bureaucracy. Madison: Institution for Research on Poverty, University of Wisconsin.

Lipsky, Michael. 1980. *Street Level Bureaucracy: Dilemmas of the Individual in Public Services*. New York: Russell Sage Foundation.

Livingston, Julie. 2005. *Debility and Moral Imagination in Botswana*. Bloomington: Indiana University Press.

Lock, Margaret. 2003. *Twice Dead: Organ Transplants and the Reinvention of Death*. Berkeley: University of California Press.

Luborsky, Mark R. 1994. "The Cultural Adversity of Physical Disability: Erosion of Full Adult Personhood." *Journal of Aging Studies* 8 (3):239–253.

Marcoux, Jean-Sebastien. 2001. "The 'Casser Maison' Ritual: Constructing the Self by Emptying the Home." *Journal of Material Culture* 6:213–235.

Marx, Karl. 1976. *Capital: A Critique of Political Economy*. Translated by Ben Fowkes. 4th ed. Vol. 1. New York: Penguin Books. Original edition, 1867.

Mattingly, Cheryl. 2014. *Moral Laboratories: Family Peril and the Struggle for a Good Life*. Berkeley: University of California Press.

Mauss, Marcel. 1979a. "A Category of the Human Mind: The Notion of Person, the Notion of 'Self.'" In *Sociology and Psychology: Essays*, edited by Ben Brewster, 59–94. London: Routledge and Kegan Paul. Original edition, 1935.

Mauss, Marcel. 1979b. "The Notion of Body Techniques." In *Sociology and Psychology: Essays*, edited by Ben Brewster, 97–123. London: Routledge and Kegan Paul. Original edition, 1935.

Mauss, Marcel. 1990. *The Gift*. Translated by W. D. Halls. London: Routledge. Original edition, 1924.

McKinnon, Susan, and Fenella Cannell, eds. 2013. *Vital Relations: Modernity and the Persistent Life of Kinship*. Santa Fe: School for Advanced Research Advanced Seminar Series.

McLean, Athena. 2007. *The Person in Dementia: A Study in Nursing Home Care in the US*. Peterborough: Broadview Press.

Meyer, Patti. 2015. "Relations of Care: The Contexts for Immigrant Care Workers in Northern Italy." *Anthropology of Work Review* 36 (1):2–12.

Minkler, Meredith, and Carroll L. Estes, eds. 1991. *Critical Perspectives on Aging: The Political and Moral Economy of Growing Old*. New York: Routledge.

Mishel, Lawrence, Josh Bivens, Elise Gould, and Heidi Shierholz. 2012. *The State of Working America*. 12th ed. Ithaca, NY: Cornell University Press.

Mittal, Vikas, Jules Rosen, and Carrie Leana. 2009. "A Dual-Driver Model of Retention and Turnover in the Direct Care Workforce." *The Gerontologist* 49 (5):623–634.

Mol, Annemarie. 2002. *The Body Multiple: Ontology in Medical Practice*. Durham, NC: Duke University Press.

Mol, Annemarie. 2008. *The Logic of Care: Health and the Problem of Patient Choice*. London: Routledge.

Mol, Annemarie, Ingunn Moser, and Jeanette Pols, eds. 2010a. *Care in Practice: On Tinkering in Clinics, Homes and Farms*. Bielefeld: Transcript Verlag.

Mol, Annemarie, Ingunn Moser, and Jeanette Pols. 2010b. "Care: Putting Practice into Theory." In *Care in Practice: On Tinkering in Clinics, Homes and Farms*, edited by Annemarie Mol, Ingunn Moser, and Jeanette Pols, 7–20. Bielefeld: Transcript Verlag.

Morris, Lisa. 2009. "Quits and Job Changes Among Home Care Workers in Maine: The Role of Wages, Hours and Benefits." The *Gerontologist* 49 (5):635–650.

Morrow-Howell, Nancy, James Hinterlong, and Michael Sherraden, eds. 2001. *Productive Aging: Concepts and Challenges*. Baltimore, MD: Johns Hopkins University Press.

Muehlebach, Andrea. 2012. *The Moral Neoliberal: Welfare and Citizenship in Italy*. Chicago: University of Chicago Press.

Mullings, Leith. 1997. *On Our Own Terms: Race, Class, and Gender in the Lives of African American Women*. New York: Routledge.

Mullings, Leith, and Alaka Wali. 2001. *Stress and Resilience: The Social Context of Reproduction in Central Harlem*. New York: Kluwer Academic/Plenum Publishers.

Nadasen, Premilla. 2016. *Household Workers Unite: The Untold Story of African American Women Who Built a Movement*. Boston: Beacon Press.

National Center for Children in Poverty. 2015. "Measuring Poverty." Columbia University Mailman School of Public Health. www.nccp.org.

Newman, Katherine S. 2001. "Hard Times on 125th Street: Harlem's Poor Confront Welfare Reform." *American Anthropologist* 103 (3):762–778.

Nicolaisen, Ida. 1995. "Persons and Nonpersons: Disability and Personhood Among the Punan Bah of Central Borneo." In *Disability and Culture*, edited by Benedicte Ingstad and Susan Reynolds Whyte, 38–55. Berkeley: University of California Press.

Ochs, Elinor, and Bambi Schieffelin. 1984. "Language Acquisition and Socialization." In *Culture Theory: Essays on Mind, Self and Emotion*, edited by Richard Shweder and Robert LeVine, 276–320. New York: Cambridge University Press.

Ochs, Elinor, and Bambi Schieffelin. 2001. "Language Acquisition and Socialization: Three Developmental Stories and Their Implications." In *Linguistic Anthropology: A Reader*, edited by Alessandro Duranti. Cambridge Cambridge University Press.

Office of Policy and Planning Research. 1965. The Negro Family: The Case for National Action. Washington, DC: US Department of Labor.

Olson, Karen, and Linda Shopes. 1991. "Crossing Boundaries: Building Bridges: Doing Oral History among Working-Class Women and Men." In *Women's Words: The Feminist Practice of Oral History*, edited by Sherna Berger Gluck and Daphne Patai. New York: Routledge.

Parreñas, Rhacel Salazar. 2001. *Servants of Globalization*. Palo Alto, CA: Stanford University Press.

Parreñas, Rhacel Salazar. 2005. *Children of Global Migration: Transnational Families and Gendered Woes*. Palo Alto, CA: Stanford University Press.

Parrott, Sharon, and Arloc Sherman. 2007. "TANF's Results are More Mixed than Is Often Understood." *Journal of Policy Analysis and Management* 26 (2):374–381.

Perry, Tam E. 2014a. "Moving as a Gift: Relocation in Older Adulthood." *Journal of Aging Studies* 31:1–9.

Perry, Tam E. 2014b. "The Rite of Relocation: Social and Material Transformations in the Midwestern United States." *Signs and Society* 2 (1):28–55.

PHI. 2015. Paying the Price: How Poverty Wages Undermine Home Care in America. New York: PHI.

PHI. 2016. U.S. Home Care Workers: Key Facts. Bronx, NY: PHInational.

PHI. 2017. "Issues: Advancing Quality Care When America Needs It Most." www.phinational.org.

Piven, Frances Fox, and Richard Cloward. 1993. *Regulating the Poor: The Functions of Public Welfare*. New York: Vintage Books.

Polanyi, Karl. 1944. *The Great Transformation*. Boston: Beacon Press.

Pollard, Leslie J. 1981. "Aging and Slavery: A Gerontological Perspective." *Journal of Negro History* 66 (3):228–234.

Poo, Ai-Jen. 2015. *The Age of Dignity: Preparing for the Elder Boom in a Changing America*. New York: New Press.

Povinelli, Elizabeth. 2002. *The Cunning of Recognition*. Durham, NC: Duke University Press.

Povinelli, Elizabeth. 2006. *Empire of Love: Toward a Theory of Intimacy, Genealogy and Carnality*. Durham, NC: Duke University Press.

Povinelli, Elizabeth, and Kim Turcot DiFrusca. 2012. "A Conversation with Elizabeth A. Povinelli." *Trans-Scripts* 2:76–90.

Radin, Margaret. 1982. "Property and Personhood." *Stanford Law Review* 34 (5):957–1015.

Ralph, Laurence. 2014. *Renegade Dreams: Living Through Injury in Gangland Chicago*. Chicago: University of Chicago Press.

Rapp, Rayna. 2000. *Testing Women, Testing the Fetus: The Social Impact of Amniocentesis in America*. New York: Routledge.

Rasmussen, Susan. 2012. "A Little to One Side: Caregiving Spatial Seclusion and Spiritual Border-Crossing in Frail Old Age Among the Tuareg (Kel Tamajaq)." *Anthropology and Aging Quarterly* 33 (4):130–141.

Reaves, Erica L., and MaryBeth Musumeci. 2015. Medicaid and Long-Term Services and Supports: A Primer. Menlo Park, CA: Kaiser Family Foundation.

Relations, Chicago Commission on Race. 1922. *The Negro in Chicago: A Study of Race Relations and a Race Riot*. Chicago: University of Chicago Press.

Riles, Annalise. 2006. *Documents: Artifacts of Modern Knowledge*. Ann Arbor: University of Michigan Press.

Robbins, Jessica. n.d. "Expanding Personhood beyond Remembered Selves: The Sociality of Memory and an Alzheimer's Center in Poland."

Robbins, Jessica. 2013. "Personhood in Places: Aging, Memory and Relatedness in Postsocialist Poland." PhD dissertation, Anthropology, University of Michigan.

Roberts, Dorothy. 1997. *Killing the Black Body*. New York: Pantheon Books.

Rollins, Judith. 1985. *Between Women: Domestics and Their Employers*. Philadelphia: Temple University Press.

Rollins, Judith. 1997. "Invisibility, Consciousness of the Other, *Ressentiment*." In *Situated Lives: Gender and Culture in Everyday Life*, edited by Louise Lamphere, Helena Ragone, and Patricia Zavella, 255–270. New York: Routledge.

Romero, Mary. 2016. *Maid in the U.S.A.* 10th anniversary edition. New York: Routledge.

Rowe, John W., and Robert Kahn. 1998. *Successful Aging*. New York: Pantheon Books.

Rubin, Gayle. 1975. "The Traffic in Women: Notes on the 'Political Economy' of Sex." In *Toward an Anthropology of Women*, edited by Rayna Reiter, 157–210. New York: Monthly Review Press.

Sacks, Karen Brodkin. 1989. "Introduction." In *My Troubles Are Going to Have Trouble with Me*, edited by Karen Brodkin Sacks and Dorothy Remy, 1–14. New Brunswick, NJ: Rutgers University Press.

Salmond, Anne. 2014. "Tears of Rangi: Water, Power and People in New Zealand." *Hau: Journal of Ethnographic Theory* 4 (3):285–309.

Sassen, Saskia. 2006. "Global Cities and Survival Circuits." In *Global Dimensions of Gender and Carework*, edited by Mary K. Zimmerman, Jacqueline S. Litt, and Christine E. Bose, 30–39. Palo Alto, CA: Stanford University Press.

Scheper-Hughes, Nancy. 1993. *Death Without Weeping: The Violence of Everyday Life in Brazil*. Berkeley: University of California Press.

Schneider, David M. 1968. *American Kinship: A Cultural Account*. Chicago: University of Chicago Press.

Schneider, David M. 1984. *A Critique of the Study of Kinship*. Ann Arbor: University of Michigan Press.

Seaman, Aaron T. 2016. "Figuring Families: Caregiving in the Midst of Alzheimer's Disease." PhD dissertation, Comparative Human Development, University of Chicago.

Shever, Elana. 2010. "Engendering the Company: Corporate Personhood and the 'Face' of an Oil Company in Metropolitan Buenos Aires." *PoLAR: Political and Legal Anthropology Review* 33 (1):26–46.

Shever, Elana. 2013. "'I am a Petroleum Product': Making Kinship Work on the Patagonian Frontier." In *Vital Relations: Modernity and the Persistent Life of Kinship*, edited by Susan McKinnon and Fenella Cannell, 85–107. Sante Fe, NM: School for Advanced Research.

Shield, Renee Rose. 1990. "Liminality in an American Nursing Home: The Endless Transition." In *The Cultural Context of Aging: Worldwide Perspectives*, edited by Jay Sokolovsky. Westport, CT: Bergin and Garvey.

Simic, Andrei. 1990. "Aging, World View, and Intergenerational Relations in America and Yugoslavia." In *The Cultural Context of Aging: Worldwide Perspectives*, edited by Jay Sokolovsky, 89–107. Westport, CT: Bergin and Garvey.

Sinclair, Upton. 1906. *The Jungle*. New York: Doubleday.

Skocpol, Theda. 1995. *Protecting Soldiers and Mothers: The Political Origins of Social Policy in the United States*. Cambridge, MA: Harvard University Press.

Smith Rolston, Jessica. 2014. *Mining Coal and Undermining Gender*. New Brunswick, NJ: Rutgers University Press.

Social Security Administration. 2006. Facts and Figures About Social Security. Washington, DC: Office of Policy; Office of Research, Evaluation, and Statistics.

Solari, Cinzia. 2006. "Professionals and Saints: How Immigrant Careworkers Negotiate Gender Identities at Work." *Gender and Society* 20:301–331.

Stacey, Clare L. 2011. *The Caring Self: The Work Experiences of Home Care Aides*. Ithaca, NY: Cornell University Press.

Stack, Carol. 1996. *Call to Home*. New York: Basic Books.

State of Illinois. 1999. Community Care Program. In *89.II.240*. Springfield: Joint Committee on Administrative Rules.

State of Illinois. 2016. Home Health, Home Services, and Home Nursing Agency Licensing Act. in *210 ILCS 55*. Springfield: Legislative Information System.

Steinem, Gloria. 1987. *Moving Beyond Words: Rage, Sex, Power, Money, Muscles: Breaking Boundaries of Gender*. New York: Simon & Schuster.

Stern, Stephanie M. 2009. "Residential Protectionism and the Legal Mythology of Home." *Michigan Law Review* 1–7 (7):1093–1144.

Stevenson, Lisa. 2014. *Life Beside Itself: Imagining Care in the Canadian Arctic*. Berkeley: University of California Press.

Stoler, Ann Laura. 2010. *Carnal Knowledge and Imperial Power*. 2nd ed. Berkeley: University of California Press.

Strathern, Marilyn. 1988. *The Gender of the Gift: Problems with Women and Problems with Society in Melanesia*. Berkeley: University of California Press.

Strathern, Marilyn. 1996. "Cutting the Network." *Journal of the Royal Anthropological Institute* 2 (3):517–535.

Strauss, Claudia. 2008. "Is Empathy Gendered, and If So, Why? An Approach from Feminist Psychological Anthropology." *Ethos* 32 (4):432–457.

Sweeney, Annie, and Jeremy Corner. 2016. "10 Shootings a Day: Complex Causes of Chicago's Spiking Violence." *Chicago Tribune*, July 3. www.chicagotribune.com.

Taylor, Charles. 1985. "The Person." In *The Category of the Person: Anthropology, Philosophy, History*, edited by Michael Carrithers, Steven Collins, and Steven Lukes, 257–281. New York: Cambridge University Press.

Taylor, Janelle S. 2008. "On Recognition, Caring, and Dementia." *Medical Anthropology Quarterly* 22 (4):313–335.

Thompson, E. P. 1963. *The Making of the English Working Class*. New York: Random House.

Thompson, E. P. 1967. "Time, Work-Discipline and Industrial Capitalism." *Past and Present* 38:56–97.

Throop, C. Jason. 2008. "On the Problem of Empathy: The Case of Yap, Federated States of Micronesia." *Ethos* 36 (4):402–426.

Throop, C. Jason. 2010. "Latitudes of Loss: On the Vicissitudes of Empathy." *American Ethnologist* 37 (4):771–782.

Throop, C. Jason. 2012. "On the Varieties of Empathic Experience." *Medical Anthropology Quarterly* 26 (3):408–430.

Throop, C. Jason, and Douglas Hollan. 2008. "Whatever Happened to Empathy." *Ethos* 36 (4):385–401.

Ticktin, Miriam. 2011. *Casualties of Care: Immigration and the Politics of Humanitarianism in France*. Berkeley: University of California Press.

Tomori, Cecilia. 2014. *Nighttime Breastfeeding: An American Cultural Dilemma*. New York: Berghahn Books.

Tronto, Joan. 1994. *Moral Boundaries: A Political Argument for an Ethic of Care*. London: Routledge.

Twigg, Julia. 2000. "Carework as a Form of Bodywork." *Aging and Society* 20:289–411.

Venkatesh, Sudhir A. 2002. *American Project: The Rise and Fall of a Modern Ghetto*. Cambridge, MA: Harvard University Press.

Venkatesh, Sudhir A. 2006. *Off the Books: The Underground Economy of the Urban Poor*. Cambridge, MA: Harvard University Press.

Vladeck, Bruce C., Paul Van de Water, and June Eichner, eds. 2007. *Strengthening Medicare's Role in Reducing Racial and Ethnic Health Disparities*. Washington, DC: National Academy of Social Insurance.

Wang, Frank T. Y. 2002. "Contesting Identity of Taiwanese Home-Care Workers: Worker, Daughter and Do-gooder?" *Journal of Aging Studies* 16:37–55.

White, Deborah Gray. 1999. *Arn't I a Woman? Female Slaves in the Plantation South*. New York: W.W. Norton.

WHO. 2015. World Report on Ageing and Health. Luxembourg: World Health Organization.

Wiles, Janine L., Annette Leibing, Nancy Guberman, Jeanne Reeve, and Ruth E. S. Allen. 2011. "The Meaning of 'Aging in Place' to Older People." *The Gerontologist* 52 (3):357–366.

Wilson, William Julius. 1996. *When Work Disappears*. New York: Random House.

Wolf-Meyer, Matthew. 2012. *The Slumbering Masses: Sleep, Medicine, and Modern American Life*. Minneapolis: University of Minnesota Press.

Wool, Zoë. 2015. *After War: The Weight of Life at Walter Reed*. Durham, NC: Duke University Press.

Yanagisako, Sylvia. 2002. *Producing Culture and Capital: Family Firms in Italy*. Princeton, NJ: Princeton University Press.

Yanagisako, Sylvia, and Jane Collier. 1987. "Toward a Unified Analysis of Gender and Kinship." In *Gender and Kinship: Essays toward a Unified Analysis*, edited by Jane Collier and Sylvia Yanagisako, 14–50. Palo Alto, CA: Stanford University Press.

Yanagisako, Sylvia, and Carol Delaney. 1995. "Naturalizing Power." In *Naturalizing Power: Essays in Feminist Cultural Analysis*, edited by Sylvia Yanagisako and Carol Delaney. New York: Routledge.

Yarris, Kristin E. 2017. *Care Across Generations: Solidarity and Sacrifice in Transnational Families*. Palo Alto, CA: Stanford University Press.

Yeates, Nicola. 2005. "A Global Political Economy of Care." *Social Policy and Society* 4 (2):227–234.

Yeates, Nicola. 2009. *Globalizing Care Economies and Migrant Workers: Explorations in Global Care Chains*. Basingstoke, UK: Palgrave Macmillan.

Yeates, Nicola. 2012. "Global Care Chains: A State-of-the-Art Review and Future Directions in Care Transnationalization Research." *Global Networks* 12 (2):135–154.

Zelizer, Viviana. 2005. *The Purchase of Intimacy*. Princeton, NJ: Princeton University Press.

Zorbaugh, Harvey W. 1929. *The Gold Coast and the Slum: A Sociological Study of Chicago's Near North Side*. Chicago: University of Chicago Press.

ABOUT THE AUTHOR

Elana D. Buch is Associate Professor of Anthropology at the University of Iowa.